Epilepsy
and
Seizures

Epilepsy and Seizures

Everything You Need to Know

Dr. Donald F. Weaver

FIREFLY BOOKS

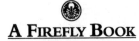

A FIREFLY BOOK

Published by Firefly Books (U.S.) Inc. 2001

Second Printing

U.S. CATALOGING IN PUBLICATION DATA

Weaver, Donald F.
   Epilepsy and seizures: everything you need to know
   / Donald F. Weaver

[168] p. : cm.
Includes bibliographic references and index.
Summary: Understanding and coping with seizure disorders.
ISBN 1-55209-452-9 (pbk.)

1. Epilepsy – Popular works. 2. Seizures – Popular works.
3. Epilepsy – Therapy.
I. Title.

618.8/5321   2001   CIP

Published in the United States in 2001 by
Firefly Books (U.S.) Inc.
P.O. Box 1338, Ellicott Station
Buffalo, New York, USA
14205

Published in Canada in 2001 by Key Porter Books Limited.

Diagrams: Theresa Sakno
Electronic formatting: Heidy Lawrance Associates

Printed and bound in Canada

Contents

For my parents

Acknowledgments

The story of the death of Charles II, in Chapter 1, is cited in *Antiepileptic Drugs*, ed. G.H. Glaser, M.D., J.K. Penry, M.D. and D.M Woodbury, Ph.D. (New York: Raven, 1980).

My thanks to Marjorie Rider for the many long hours she spent helping me prepare the manuscript for this book. I am also grateful to the directors and members of Epilepsy Kingston for sharing their insiders' perspective on living with this difficult condition.

D.W.

Introduction

Epilepsy is like no other medical condition. For many people it is a chronic yet intermittent disorder; they may go months or even years without a seizure. For others it begins in childhood and persists, with little relief, for a lifetime. Either way, people with epilepsy don't know when their next seizure will occur – maybe in two minutes, maybe next year. Epilepsy is not like the dementia of Alzheimer's, which occurs mainly in the elderly. It is not like heart attack or stroke, both of which strike acutely and may never happen again. Epilepsy is unique.

Most people with epileptic seizures have seen many physicians and neurologists, and have tried many drugs and combinations of drugs. They have been offered a great deal of advice about their epilepsy, some of it right, much of it wrong. They have joined epilepsy associations that provide them with a constant flow of information in comprehensive pamphlets and newsletters. And for those with Internet connections there are many websites. Because information about new research and medical advances in the field is so widely available, many people with epilepsy are extremely knowledgeable about their disorder, and expect to take an active part in decisions about their treatment.

The aim of this book is to provide an overview of all the important current medical knowledge of epilepsy, to help you make informed decisions – for yourself or for a family member

– about the healthcare that is best for you. Patients and their families were widely consulted during the preparation of the book, and the questions they most commonly ask have all been answered in these pages, to the best of my ability. The case studies describe real people with real problems (though their names have been changed to protect their privacy). In particular, take-home points have been included at the ends of the chapters to provide quick, reliable summaries of the facts that people with epilepsy most need to know.

ONE

Epilepsy through the Ages

The history of epilepsy is a history of evil spirits and curses, of medical ignorance and human suffering, of mysticism and charlatanism. In times past, the illness was thought to be a "sacred disease" caused by gods or devils who wanted to punish or take revenge on mortals. The word "epilepsy" is derived from the Greek *epilambanein* (to take or seize), and the belief that a powerful spirit takes over or seizes the patient's brain is reflected in the term "seizure" itself. In the ancient world, *trephining* (also called *trepanning*) was the usual treatment: holes were drilled in the patient's skull to release the demons.

The Greeks and Romans gained new insights into epilepsy. Between 400 BC and 200 AD, the physicians Hippocrates, Aretaeus, Celsus and Plinius all provided careful descriptions of major and minor seizures. Hippocrates even recognized that seizures originated in the brain. Despite this relative enlightenment as to the condition's cause, the treatments of the time continued to be gruesome and at times grotesque. Some people believed that drinking the warm blood of a freshly slain gladiator or wearing a necklace made from the penis of a seal would cure the seizures. Others drank revolting mixtures containing mistletoe, dog urine or human bile.

1

What is epilepsy?

Epilepsy is not a disease. Rather, it is a symptom originating in the brain. This complex organ is composed of between ten billion and one hundred billion small structural units called brain cells. Brain cells communicate with each other by means of tiny bursts of electrical activity. Sometimes a group of brain cells has an unexpected, erratic electrical discharge. This event produces a *seizure*. Someone who has multiple seizures is said to have *epilepsy*, which is defined as a functional disorder of the brain caused by sudden, brief malfunctions. These malfunctions may cause uncontrollable shaking (convulsions). They may also cause loss of awareness, confusion or even disturbance of the senses (visual and aural hallucinations, phantom odors, etc.).

The aim of these was always the same: to drive out the evil spirits that were tormenting the afflicted person.

During the Middle Ages, beliefs about epilepsy continued to be primitive and cruel. Many sufferers were punished rather than treated; some were burned at the stake. The illness was considered to be a form of madness, and treatments offered by medieval doctors were no less violent than those of the ancients. The following description of the death of King Charles II is typical of how the aristocracy (who had access to the best physicians) were treated for their seizures. The king had a convulsion while he was being shaved, and a dozen or so physicians were called in to treat him.

He was bled to the extent of 1 pint from his right arm. Next, his shoulder was incised and "cupped," depriving him of another 8 oz. of blood. After an emetic and 2 purgatives, he was given an enema containing antimony, sacred bitters, rock salt, mallow leaves, violets, beet root, camomile flowers, fennel seed, linseed, cinnamon, cardamom seed, saffron, and aloes. The enema was repeated in 2 hours and another purgative given. The king's head was shaved and a blister raised on his scalp. A sneezing powder of hellebore root and one of cowslip flowers were administered "to strengthen the king's brain." Soothing drinks of barley water, licorice, and sweet almond were given, as well as extracts of mint, thistle leaves, rue, and angelica. For external treatment, a plaster of Burgundy pitch and pigeon dung was applied to the king's feet.

After continued bleeding and purging, to which were added melon seeds, manna, slippery elm, black cherry water, and dissolved pearls, the king's condition did not improve and, as an emergency measure, 40 drops of human skull extract were given to allay convulsions. A rallying dose of Raleigh's antidote was also given. This contained an enormous amount of herbs and animal extracts. Finally bezoar stone was given. As the king's condition grew increasingly worse, the grand finale of Raleigh's antidote, pearl julep, and ammonia water was forced down the dying king's throat.

Epilepsy in the Modern Era

A better understanding of epilepsy began to emerge in the second half of the eighteenth century. Samuel Tissot's *Traité de l'epilésie* (1770) reflected extensive and accurate observation of the disorder, and by the mid-1800s, pathologists such as Wilhelm Sommer had published descriptions of the brain changes associated with the condition. Fifty years later the British neurologist Hughlings Jackson provided a modern definition of a seizure, which helped to move epilepsy out of the domain of the psychiatrist into that of the neurologist. The myth that epilepsy was a form of insanity was slowly being disproved. A short time later another neurologist, Sir William Richard Gowers, provided meticulous descriptions of seizure types.

In 1857 a new treatment of epilepsy was introduced, representing a quantum leap forward for the patient. Sir Charles Locock, a physician to Queen Victoria, theorized that epilepsy

What causes epilepsy?

Malfunction of brain activity begins with an injury, or *insult*. When brain cells are injured, by whatever cause (birth trauma, stroke, head trauma or brain tumors, for example), they respond in one of two ways. They may quit functioning altogether, as in the paralysis associated with stroke; or they may "overfunction," producing convulsions. Anyone, at any age, can have an epileptic seizure, if the brain is influenced sufficiently by genetic predisposition, injury or disease. It can happen to a professional athlete or a quadriplegic confined to a wheelchair. The seizure varies from person to person, depending on where in the brain it originates. However, all epilepsy sufferers have one thing in common: the knowledge that seizures are unpredictable, frequently striking like a bolt of lightning from a cloudless sky.

was due to excessive sexuality, and in an attempt to control this supposed problem he administered sodium bromide to seizure patients. These people experienced a significant improvement. Although we now recognize that this was due, not to any influence on their sexuality, but to the activity of sodium bromide on chloride channels within the brain, it nevertheless was the first time epilepsy sufferers had been given a medication that worked. In the early 1900s, two other drugs, phenobarbital and phenytoin, joined the ranks of effective therapeutics. For people with epilepsy, the modern era had definitely created new hope!

Almost As Common As Headache

After headache, epilepsy is the neurologic disorder most often seen by physicians. In terms of *prevalence* (defined as the proportion of active cases within a particular population at any one time), epilepsy is extremely common – it occurs in approximately one percent of the general population. It does, however, vary from country to country, depending upon socioeconomic conditions. In developed countries its prevalence is lower (around 0.5 to 0.8 percent). If one of the parents has epilepsy, the risk of a child developing epilepsy is 4 to 5 percent. This risk is elevated to 6 to 8 percent if any of the following is also present: a sibling with seizures, both parents with seizures, a history of seizures in one or more grandparents or an abnormal electroencephalogram (see Chapter 4). In developing countries the proportion of active cases is 1.3 percent, and it may be as high as 4 percent in certain African countries. This high figure arises from the greater incidence of birth trauma, infections in the newborn and head trauma.

Incidence, as opposed to prevalence, is the annual rate of appearance of new cases. It is usually expressed as the number of new cases per hundred thousand population per year. Once again, there is a difference between developed and developing countries. In developed countries the incidence is approximately 50 cases per 100,000 population per year. In developing countries the incidence is approximately 160 cases per 100,000 population per year. In a large North American city with a population of approximately two million people, four new cases of epilepsy will be diagnosed each and every day.

An estimated 1.8 million people in North America suffer from epilepsy. This is an enormous proportion of the population, far exceeding the numbers with multiple sclerosis, muscular dystrophy, cerebral palsy or any other relatively well known neurologic problems. An even greater number of people (between 5 and 9 percent of the general population) have at least one seizure in their lifetime. However, only a condition involving *multiple* seizures is defined as epilepsy, and a person who has experienced one seizure does not necessarily have epilepsy. A single seizure may result from a variety of medical conditions. Simple febrile (fever) convulsions are the most common cause of isolated seizures in children under age eight.

People with epilepsy know how widespread the condition

is, and will not be surprised to learn that it has a very significant social and economic impact. They are already aware of the personal toll it can take.

Seizures and Genetic Factors

Given certain conditions, absolutely anybody can experience a seizure. Why, then, do some people experience seizures frequently and other people not at all? The answer to this question lies in the complex interrelationship between genetics (or heredity) and acquired factors.

There are a small number of people with epilepsy whose seizures arise from a chromosome abnormality or an inherited genetic trait. However, these causes account for less than 5 percent of all people with seizure disorders. There are also well over a hundred different inherited disorders involving chemical or structural abnormalities in the brain that can directly lead to epilepsy. However, many of these disorders are rare to the point of obscurity, and more than a third of people afflicted by them also have severe mental retardation.

What about the 95 percent of people with seizures who have neither a directly inherited nor a genetic form of epilepsy? Are genetic factors involved with these people as well? Probably.

Studies have been made of veterans of several wars, including World War I, the Korean War and the Vietnam War. In one study, fifty soldiers who had been shot in the head and later developed epilepsy were compared to fifty soldiers who had been shot in the head but did not develop epilepsy. The results were interesting. Soldiers who developed epilepsy tended to have relatives who had epilepsy, while soldiers who did not develop epilepsy tended not to have any people with epilepsy in their extended family. It appears that we inherit our family's *seizure threshold*. We may inherit a predisposition toward epilepsy, but whether or not we develop seizures may depend on what triggering events – such as brain trauma or infection – we later encounter.

Epilepsy in Childhood

Epilepsy can appear at any age. There is a peak of incidence, in most countries, during the childhood years; 50 to 60 percent of epilepsy begins prior to age 16. (It's important to remember, though, that between 2 and 4 percent of children experience febrile convulsions, which do not necessarily carry an increased risk of subsequent epilepsy.) Epilepsy most often appears in the first two years of life, or in the years surrounding puberty. The reasons for the onset of epilepsy in childhood are multiple, and include difficult birth, childhood infections and childhood head trauma.

Angela remembers the day when she learned that her son had epilepsy. "I was horrified. I thought he must have something terribly wrong with his brain. My grandmother had told me when I was a little girl that people with epilepsy eventually go insane. This is wrong – quite wrong – as I soon learned. His seizures were controlled with drugs and he is doing well in school. But even though he hasn't had a seizure in 18 months, not a day goes by that I don't worry about him having another one."

Epilepsy in Adults

Although epilepsy can begin at any age, the first seizure is least likely to occur in young and middle-aged adults, particularly between the ages of 30 and 50. However, since 60 percent of epilepsy begins early and persists into adulthood, many adults do have epilepsy.

Epilepsy in the Elderly

The likelihood of a first seizure occurring increases again, in most countries, once people are elderly. This results from the increasing likelihood of strokes and certain other brain injuries at this extreme of age. The rate of new cases in people between the ages of 70 and 80 is dramatic – sometimes as high as one in a thousand in a given year. Recent studies suggest that the peak in young children has declined in recent years, but that the peak in the elderly has actually risen. This is significant because the average age of our population is increasing, and the treatment of seizures in elderly people, who may be more sensitive to the medications required, can be difficult.

Take-home points
- The history of epilepsy is long and filled with prejudice.
- Epilepsy is extremely common, affecting approximately one percent of the population.
- The onset of epilepsy is more common in young children and the elderly than in young or middle-aged adults.

TWO

The Biology of Epilepsy

Epilepsy is a condition of the brain. When you experience a seizure, its nature and symptoms depend on its point of origin within your brain. Accordingly, to understand seizures it is first necessary to understand a little about the structure and function of the brain.

The brain controls how we think, feel, move, see and hear. Although it weighs less than 3 pounds (1.1 to 1.4 kg), the human brain is the home of all of our memories, thoughts, desires, lusts, ambitions and dreams. It is what makes each of us unique; it is responsible for our idealistic aspirations and our primitive urges, for our greatest achievements and our most humbling failures. Yet despite its importance and its lofty tasks, the brain is particularly unprepossessing: it's gray, and it has the shape of a wrinkled walnut and the consistency of jelly.

Structurally, the human brain is composed of billions of microscopic units called nerve cells or *neurons*, each of which is capable of generating and transmitting electrical signals. A nerve cell consists of three main regions: *cell body*, *dendrite* and *axon*. The cell body contains the machinery necessary for maintaining the health and well-being of the nerve cell. The dendrite receives electrical information from adjacent nerve cells, in electrical signals that travel down the axon of the nerve cell. Nerve cells do not touch each other, but are separated by a gap called a *synapse*. The electrical signal crosses the gap, transmitting information from one neuron to the next, via a chemical messenger called a *neurotransmitter*; the neurotransmitter is released by the sending cell, and when it diffuses to the receiving cell it sets off the electrical signal there. Neurotransmitters may be either *excitatory*, causing a spread of electrical excitation to an adjacent nerve cell, or *inhibitory*, tending to decrease electrical excitability in an adjacent nerve cell.

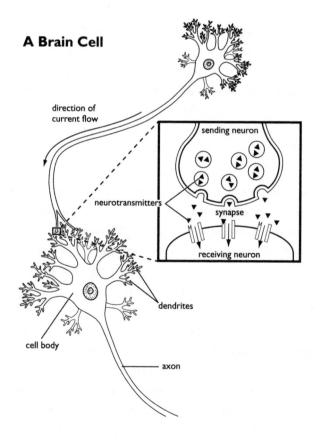

A Brain Cell

direction of
current flow

sending neuron

neurotransmitters

synapse

receiving neuron

dendrites

cell body

axon

What is a seizure?

A seizure is a single event. It is an abnormal and excessive discharge of electrical activity from a collection of neurons. This discharge is accompanied by some behavioral change in the individual. Changes may be dramatic, or may be quite subtle; some are detectable only through specialized tests, such as a precise measurement of reaction time. Epilepsy is the disorder experienced by people who have multiple seizures; it is a chronic condition characterized by a predisposition to recurrent, usually spontaneous seizures.

In addition to nerve cells, there is another group of cells called *glial cells*. These are support cells, which carry out functions such as the removal of waste materials generated by the very active nerve cells.

These two types of cells constitute the bulk of the brain. Together they also form the other gross anatomical structures of the human nervous system, which is divided into two sections: *central* and *peripheral*.

The central nervous system consists of the spinal cord and brain. The spinal cord, which runs from the base of the brain down to about hip level, is approximately two feet long and acts primarily as a conduit carrying sensory and motor information to and from the brain.

The peripheral nervous system extends throughout the body, right down to fingers and toes. It delivers sensory information to the central nervous system, and carries motor information back to the muscles. For example, when a hand is placed on a hot stove, the sensory information (heat and pain perception) is carried to the central nervous system, and the motor response (to move the hand off the stove) is transmitted from the central nervous system back to the muscles of the arm and hand.

A Quick Tour of the Brain

The brain has two main parts: the *brain stem* and the two *cerebral hemispheres*. Located behind the brain stem is the *cerebellum*, a diminutive but very important structure. It is responsible for coordination of movement – for example, drunks stagger because their cerebellums are not working properly. The cerebellum is quite sensitive to drugs and chemicals, with the result that some people react to medications as if they were toxic.

A Cross-Section of the Brain

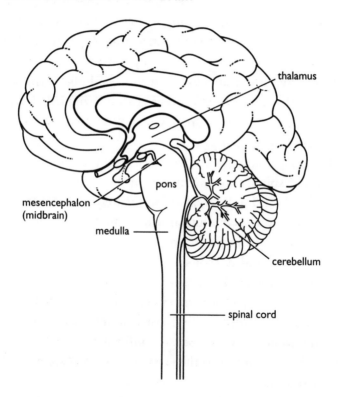

The brain stem itself is composed of the *medulla oblongata, pons* and *mesencephalon*. The medulla oblongata is an inch of vital brain located just above the spinal cord; it controls heart rate, blood pressure, breathing, talking, swallowing and vomiting. Injury to the medulla usually results in death within minutes. Just above the medulla is the pons (Latin for "bridge"), so named because it's between the cerebellum and the cerebral hemispheres. Above the pons is the midbrain or mesencephalon, which, despite being the smallest segment of the brain stem, is the most sophisticated. Four small *colliculli* ("little hills") located on the back portion of the midbrain permit hearing and seeing.

The midbrain is connected to the cerebral hemispheres via the *diencephalon*. The two most important structures within the diencephalon are the *thalamus* and the *hypothalamus*. The cerebral hemispheres rest on the thalamus, which acts as a central station relaying all sensory information from the body to the cerebral hemispheres. The hypothalamus is involved in regulating most of the body's critical activities. It controls water balance, food intake, body temperature, sexual rhythms and the *autonomic nervous system*, and regulates complex states such as hunger, anger and placidity, while orchestrating the behaviors that accompany emotional states. (The autonomic nervous system is a branch of the peripheral nervous system extending into internal organs such as heart, lungs and stomach.)

Above the diencephalon, at the base of the cerebral hemispheres, is a group of structures called the basal ganglia, which facilitate the performance of learned repetitive motor activities such as walking or riding a bicycle. Damage to the basal ganglia can lead to disorders such as Huntington's or Parkinson's disease.

Each cerebral hemisphere contains four lobes: frontal, parietal, temporal and occipital. The frontal lobes are the primary area for motor movement, with each side controlling the opposite side of the body. Thus injury to the frontal lobe of the right hemisphere causes paralysis (motor weakness) on the left side of the body. The parietal lobes are the primary areas for sensation, and injury to one of these areas causes hemi-anesthesia (inability to feel sensations) in the opposite side of the body. The occipital lobes are the primary areas for vision, and damage can result in a loss of vision, though sometimes only in certain directions. The function of the temporal lobes is not so clear-cut or well understood, but damage can result in memory problems, auditory hallucinations, psychotic behavior, changes in vision, disturbances in time perception, balance problems, inability to distinguish between various sounds, speech difficulties and inability to recognize qualities in music.

The Lobes of the Brain

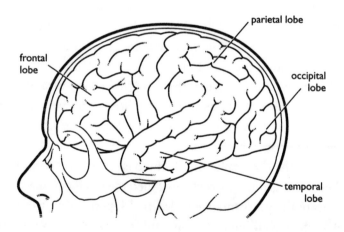

Where Seizures Take Place

Understanding the brain's anatomy often helps people with epilepsy to gain insight into the nature of their seizures. Seizures do not arise from abnormalities of the peripheral nervous system or the spinal cord, and they cannot be treated by manipulations of the spinal cord. Typically, seizures arise within the cerebrum, from electrical misfirings that are usually traceable to some form of injury to one or more of the brain's lobes. The temporal lobe is the area where seizures seem to originate most often.

The area of the brain where a seizure begins is called the *focus*, and this is the location of the malfunctioning, electrically excitable neurons. The exact location of this focus influences the nature of the seizure. For example, if the focus is in one of the motor portions of the frontal lobe, the seizure may start with shaking of the opposite side of the body. If it arises from the occipital lobe, the seizure may begin with some sort of visual abnormality, such as a hallucination. A malfunction in the temporal lobe may cause a seizure beginning with difficulties of speech.

The Focus and the Spread

Most people know that the brain is made up of *gray matter* (the term is sometimes loosely used to mean intelligence). However, each structure of the brain, such as the frontal lobe, has both gray and white matter in its composition: the gray is the cell bodies of the neurons, and the white is the axons of the neurons, which are coated with insulation made from fat, and thus appear white. Think of the brain as an electrical system. The electrical boxes containing the switches and breakers are like the cell bodies of the gray matter; the wires leading away from these electrical boxes, covered with insulation, are like the fat-coated axons of the white matter.

Epilepsy is a disorder of the gray matter only. The small damaged area of gray matter, called the *focus*, is abnormally electrically excitable. When this focus discharges its electrical activity suddenly and unexpectedly, the result is a seizure. The first symptoms are directly related to the location of the focus but, since the brain is a highly integrated network of electrical systems, the electrical activity can spread rapidly throughout the brain. As it does so, the symptoms of the seizure become more pronounced and more dramatic.

Consider, for example, the case of someone with a seizure focus in the motor portion of the frontal-lobe gray matter, affecting a small area on the left side of the brain. When the focus fires, the person may experience rhythmic shaking of the index finger of the right hand, which may persist for seconds or minutes. As the electrical activity spreads along normal pathways from the focus into the rest of the brain, the rhythmical shaking will also spread: from the finger to the hand, then to the forearm and to the entire arm. It may spread over the whole right side of the body, and may ultimately affect the entire body, as the electrical activity spreads to both sides of the brain. This would then culminate in a *generalized seizure*. This progression of seizure activity – like a forest fire spreading from tree to tree – is referred to as a *Jacksonian march*, after the British neurologist who first described it.

How the Electrical Activity Spreads within the Brain
Electrical activity spreads along the surface of the brain cell by the sequential opening of tiny pores. These pores, called *sodium channels* and *calcium channels*, permit small charged particles of sodium and calcium (ions) to enter the nerve cell. A wave of ions entering a nerve cell sequentially along the surface of the cell leads to the spread of electrical excitation. Drugs that block either the sodium channel or the calcium channel can therefore decrease the spread of abnormal electrical activity within the brain (see Chapter 5).

Types of Brain Injury Leading to Seizures

As explained earlier, when neurons are injured they can respond in one of two ways: they can cease to function, leading to paralysis, or overfunction, creating an electrical excitability and thus seizures. Both loss of function and overfunctioning can result from the same injury. For example, when a stroke (see below) affects a group of neurons, some (at the center of the stroke) may stop functioning while others (in the periphery of the stroke) overfunction and cause a seizure.

In approximately 65 percent of people with epilepsy, the event that first produced an electrically excitable focus, causing the seizures, is never discovered. In the other 35 percent, a cause can be pinpointed. Strokes and other conditions causing altered blood supply to the brain account for 15 percent of all cases of epilepsy. Developmental factors (injuries before or during birth) or genetic factors account for another 5 to 6 percent, and injury to the brain in the form of trauma produces about 4 percent. A further 4 percent are caused by brain tumors, either benign or malignant, while infection of the brain or the membranes that surround it produces another 3 percent. Degenerative diseases of the brain, such as Alzheimer's disease, produce 1 to 2 percent. Drugs and other substances, such as alcohol, account for the final 2 percent.

Stroke

Stroke is a leading identified cause of epilepsy. A stroke is defined as the sudden onset of a brain dysfunction arising from an abrupt alteration in the blood supply to the brain. An *ischemic* stroke occurs when an artery supplying blood to the brain is suddenly blocked. A *hemorrhagic* stroke is produced when an artery supplying blood to the brain suddenly breaks, spilling its blood; hemorrhagic strokes can be caused by high blood pressure or by defects within the structure of the artery called *aneurysms*. In any stroke, the part of the brain that was receiving blood from the affected artery quits functioning, and if the blood supply is not restored, that part of the brain will die.

Various terms are used to describe ischemic strokes. If the signs and symptoms last less than 24 hours, the stroke is called a *transient ischemic attack* (TIA). Transient ischemic attacks are sometimes called mini-strokes. If the signs and symptoms persist longer than 24 hours, the event is called a stroke or *brain attack*. If the person is left with a major disability, the event is referred to as a major stroke or a *dense stroke*; if the resulting deficits are relatively mild, it is referred to as a minor stroke.

Stroke is the most common cause of the onset of epilepsy among people over 50, accounting for 70 to 80 percent of all cases, and in recent years it has been recognized that very small, perhaps even unrecognizable strokes are causing late-onset epilepsy in increasing numbers of people. Approximately 8 percent of stroke survivors will have seizures within two weeks following the stroke. Within two years of the stroke, 10 percent of ischemic stroke survivors and 15 to 20 percent of hemorrhagic stroke survivors will have epilepsy. The size of the stroke is a very important factor in determining the likelihood of someone developing epilepsy.

Developmental and Genetic Disorders

Developmental and genetic disorders account for the next-largest group of epilepsy sufferers. If a pregnant woman is exposed to certain infections or drugs, developmental disorders can arise as the brain is forming in the fetus. Neurons migrate within the developing fetal brain; damage during this migration process can result in brain cells not reaching their correct position, causing the development of a seizure focus.

Genetic disorders are not the same as developmental disorders; they reflect the inheritance of a predisposition from one or both parents. There are more than 141 single-gene disorders that cause brain abnormalities associated with epilepsy. Other genetic disorders are also often associated with epilepsy: for example, 10 to 15 percent of people with trisomy 21, also known as Down's syndrome, have epilepsy as well.

Brain Trauma

Brain trauma from traffic accidents, sports injuries and other violent events can also cause epilepsy. Risk-taking young men are particularly likely to develop epilepsy in this manner. The overall risk of developing epilepsy within four years of a head injury is approximately 7 percent in the civilian population and 34 percent among soldiers who suffer head injuries in combat. Of those who do develop epilepsy after head trauma, 60 percent will develop it within one year of the injury, 85 percent within two years and 98 percent within five years. The more severe the head injury, the more likely it is that epilepsy will follow, and the risk is higher with penetrating injuries such as gunshot wounds and depression fractures (in which part of the skull is driven inwards). Head injuries associated with unconsciousness lasting more than 24 hours and with bleeding into the brain are the ones most likely to lead to epilepsy.

Brain Tumors

Brain tumors are also a common cause of epilepsy. According to some studies, approximately 35 to 40 percent of people who experienced seizures and the onset of epilepsy in adulthood were ultimately diagnosed with tumors. Epilepsy can also be caused by tumors that originate elsewhere in the body but spread to the brain: for example, lung cancer caused by smoking can spread to the brain and produce recurrent seizures.

"Boy, kids can be cruel," says Claude. "It took years of people laughing at me before someone figured out what exactly my spells were. Apparently, a couple times per day I give a funny sort of laugh. I don't know I'm doing it. One of my teachers called it an evil-sounding laugh, not a happy laugh. She described it as a sinister, from-beyond-the-grave laugh. Finally, one of my pediatricians figured out that this was a problem called gelastic epilepsy. They did a CT scan and found a tumor in my head. They call it a 'hypothalamic hamartoma.'

"Apparently it's some benign tumor in the center of my brain. Since it isn't growing, the doctors have decided to leave it where it is for the time being. They have stopped my seizures with two drugs – topiramate and lamotrigine. My teacher isn't convinced, but at least the other kids don't make fun of me anymore."

Infection
Cerebral infection may be caused by bacteria, viruses, fungi or parasites. An infection that involves the brain itself is called an *encephalitis*; one that affects the membranes covering the brain is called *meningitis*. Both can produce epilepsy. The seizures may occur acutely at the time of the infection, or many years later. In the past ten years it has been realized that AIDS is a growing cause of infection-related epilepsy; in one study of 630 AIDS patients, 13 percent experienced seizures. In addition, approximately 25 percent of survivors of herpes simplex encephalitis develop epilepsy. Tuberculosis, a common cause of brain infections in developing countries, leads to epilepsy in 70 percent of surviving patients. Jakob-Creutzfeldt disease can also lead to seizures.

Cerebral Degenerative Disorders
Cerebral degeneration of the kind associated with Alzheimer's disease is being increasingly recognized as a cause of epilepsy.

Seizures are uncommon early in the course of Alzheimer's, but they occur in approximately one-third of those in the late stages of the disease. There are other, less common degenerative disorders of the brain, including rare disorders such as Pick's disease, that are also associated with seizures. On the other hand, although multiple sclerosis (MS) is a brain disorder, it is associated with epilepsy in only about 3 percent of cases. MS is a disease of white matter rather than gray matter, and it doesn't cause seizures unless the white-matter abnormality impinges directly on adjacent gray matter.

Drug and Alcohol Abuse

Many drugs can provoke seizures. Cocaine often causes seizures, and may do brain damage leading to chronic epilepsy. Amphetamines and LSD are also drugs of abuse associated with seizures. Many therapeutic drugs, including penicillin, theophylline, certain antidepressants and a variety of antipsychotic drugs, can cause isolated seizures. Even some nonprescription drugs may increase the likelihood of having seizures; antihistamines, commonly found in cold and allergy remedies, are a frequent culprit. Alcohol is likewise a major cause of drug-induced seizures; more than 15 percent of alcoholics will experience seizures, mostly in connection with alcohol withdrawal. Such seizures, also called rum fits, occur in people whose alcohol abuse is heavy and chronic. Another significant risk factor associated with heavy drinking is the high incidence of head injury in people who abuse alcohol.

Other Medical Problems Leading to Seizures

Trauma, infections and intoxications that damage brain cells are the major causes of seizures, but occasionally problems arising outside the brain are responsible. Changes in hormones and chemicals throughout the body during non-neurologic illnesses can influence the brain, which in such circumstances is simply an innocent bystander. The most frequent example is *electrolyte disturbance*, which occurs when the levels of salts in the bloodstream, such as sodium chloride, fall too low. This can happen when bodily fluids are lost through severe diarrhea or vomiting, or after extended heavy exertion. The problem of lost body fluids is widely recognized by long-distance runners and other athletes, who drink special salt-rich beverages to replenish their losses; they know that even the loss of a substantial amount of sodium chloride (plain salt) may produce seizures, although it does not lead to chronic epilepsy.

The second most important non-brain cause of seizures is the disturbed glucose metabolism associated with diabetes. Glucose is a simple sugar used by the brain as an important source of energy. To process glucose the body needs insulin, either natural or administered. Because people with diabetes have trouble keeping their glucose and insulin in balance, they sometimes have *hypoglycemia* (too little glucose) or *hyperglycemia* (too much glucose). Both extremes are associated with seizures, but the seizures stop when the glucose imbalance is corrected.

People with failing kidneys frequently have *uremia*, or increased blood levels of certain toxins that would normally be removed by the kidneys. These toxins may be associated with seizures. The problem can be corrected by dialysis or a kidney transplant.

A variety of studies suggest that seizures also occur in 2 to 33 percent of people with liver failure. The long-term use of antiseizure drugs is not required once the underlying problem has been corrected.

Finally, diseases of the thyroid or parathyroid glands may lead to seizures. In rare cases, the thyroid produces too little of a hormone called thyroxine and seizures result. Similarly, the parathyroid glands, small structures located in the neck on either side of the thyroid gland, are responsible for regulating calcium levels in the blood. If they are not functioning at full capacity, seizures may occur.

Take-home points

- Epilepsy is not a disease in itself, but a symptom.
- Epilepsy is characterized by recurrent seizures.
- A seizure is produced by an excessive electrical discharge from a collection of brain cells.
- Many types of brain injury can lead to seizures.
- In more than half of all people with recurrent seizures, no cause is ever identified.

T H R E E

*Types of
Seizures and
Epilepsy*

Your doctor may describe seizures using terms like *grand mal* or *petit mal*; *generalized*, *partial* or *complex*; *tonic*, *clonic* or *absence*. The electrical complexity of the human brain means that a wide range of seizure types is possible. Just as there are different types of seizures, so are there different types of epilepsy. But most seizures and epilepsies fit into established classification schemes, and your doctor will identify your specific type in order to establish what medications will be best for you.

Seizures can be categorized into two broad types: *partial* and *primary generalized*. Partial seizures arise from a localized seizure focus within the brain. Depending on the location of this focus, the symptoms vary widely. If the abnormal electrical activity of the partial seizure spreads to both hemispheres of the brain, it gives rise to a *secondary generalized* seizure.

Primary generalized seizures have no focal features; they are characterized from the beginning by involvement of wide areas of the brain. There are many types of generalized seizures.

A table at the end of this chapter shows the classification of seizure types, as established by the International League against Epilepsy.

Origins of Seizures

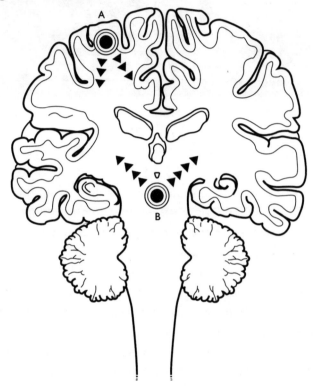

A partial seizure begins in a specialized area of the brain (A) and spreads from there. A generalized seizure (B) spreads into both hemispheres at the same time.

Partial and Secondary Generalized Seizures

Simple Partial Seizures

An older term for this type of seizure was *focal* or *local* seizure. Depending on the location of the seizure focus, simple partial seizures may manifest themselves in motor signs, such as

Simple partial seizures

Cheryl says, "My seizures aren't like anybody else's at the Epilepsy Association. I never lose awareness or consciousness with my seizures. All of a sudden, the pointer finger of my left hand will start to jump. Sometimes, that's all there is to it. Sometimes my whole left hand or arm will also shake. It never gets any worse than that. It shakes for a few minutes and then it's over. I have no control over it. Fortunately, I'm awake and alert for the whole thing."

rhythmic jerking of a hand or arm; sensory symptoms, such as abnormal sensations in part of the body; or psychic symptoms, such as hallucinations. They usually begin suddenly and last only a very short time. There is absolutely no loss of consciousness or awareness, which is why the seizures are called "simple."

During a simple partial seizure originating in the frontal lobe, someone may utter a sound, or may be unable to speak; the head or eyes may be averted to one side. Simple partial seizures of temporal-lobe origin are different, and widely variable. They may involve an unusual feeling at the top of the abdomen, hallucinations or the perception of unusual odors. Different again are simple partial seizures of parietal-lobe origin, which may involve unusual sensations or tingling, often in the face, arm or hand. Finally, simple partial seizures of occipital-lobe origin are usually associated with visual symptoms. These may be hallucinations or other distorted perceptions of light, color or patterns.

Complex Partial Seizures

Complex partial seizures are associated with an altered level of consciousness, and they have a highly variable range of symptoms. According to the textbook description, they typically begin with an unusual feeling at the top of the abdomen, just below the breastbone. Most people find it almost impossible to describe this feeling. Some call it nausea, or describe it as "like butterflies in my stomach." It appears that the English language just doesn't have a word for it – and other languages are equally lacking. The feeling rises from the upper abdomen, behind the breastbone, sometimes even into the lower face. A short time thereafter, the person's level of consciousness diminishes. During this phase, observers note that the person's eyes are open but that he or she is unresponsive. As the saying goes, "The lights are on but there's nobody home." During this blank, unresponsive staring spell, the person may carry out random, purposeless movements called *automatisms*. These movements may take the form of chewing motions or lip-smacking. Alternatively, people may play with their clothing or make picking motions in the air. Usually the seizure lasts one and a half to two minutes, but the person tends to be somewhat confused and disoriented for an additional 15 to 20 minutes, and may not fully return to normal for hours.

Lynette is 24 years old. At the age of 7, she was playing beside her house in a sandbox. A loose brick fell from the chimney, striking her in the left side of the head, causing a small area of brain damage. Her complex partial seizures began at age 17.

"I always know when I'm about to have a seizure. All of a sudden I can't speak properly. My co-workers laugh at me saying, 'There she goes getting her *mords wixed up again* – instead of *words mixed up again*.' I know the word I want to say, but I just cannot say it. Sometimes I insert another word that doesn't make sense; sometimes I insert a word that rhymes. As the seizure worsens, I completely lose my ability to speak. I simply sit there in a dreamy world. I'm aware of what's happening around me, I just can't interact with my surroundings. If someone comes into the room, I know they've entered but I can't recognize them and I certainly can't talk to them. This dreaming feeling lasts about two minutes, then I return to normal. Sometimes I continue to have speaking problems for a few minutes. Once I was completely unable to speak for about 15 minutes."

Ted developed complex partial seizures at the age of 26, 18 months after being struck in the side of the head by a hockey puck.

"My seizures start with a funny feeling at the top of my stomach. I use the word 'nausea' to describe it, but it really isn't nausea. The feeling stays there for 20 or 30 seconds, but it can last several minutes. It then starts to rise up through my body, the same weird feeling. After this, I don't know what happens. My wife says I just stop and stare. My eyes are open but I don't respond to anything. I just sit quietly. I don't shake or jerk. I sometimes make chewing motions with my mouth, but that's all. Then I wake up and feel confused and dazed, and really tired. Sometimes I sleep for four hours or so."

Barry is 20. He developed his seizures at 16. There is no history of head trauma, meningitis or injury to the brain, and no family history of seizures. The CT scan of his head is normal.

"I never know when I'm going to have a seizure. Everything I'm going to tell you about my seizures has been told to me by other people, especially my mother. Apparently my head turns to the right and my eyes roll to the right. Sometimes I get up from a seated position and walk about the room in circles, or I lie down on the floor and put my legs up in the air making bicycling motions. During this time I'm staring with a glazed expression. Then, just as suddenly as it started, the seizure ends. Almost immediately I'm right back to normal, and I don't remember anything. I really hate having these seizures. Everyone looks at me and I feel very uncomfortable. Initially everyone thought I was somehow faking, and my family doctor sent me to a psychiatrist. It took a couple of years to get these spells diagnosed as seizures."

Many people with complex partial seizures have quite peculiar symptoms. For example, they may have an olfactory hallucination, in which they perceive nonexistent odors. Others, like Barry, have peculiar behaviors which may not be recognized as epileptic, even by experienced observers. (These sensations and movements are called *auras*, and are a form of simple partial seizure.)

Complex partial seizures most frequently arise in either the temporal or frontal lobe, and there are definite differences between the two. The automatisms of a frontal-lobe complex partial seizure may include bicycling motions of the legs, or pelvic thrusting. Also, those of frontal-lobe origin tend to resolve more quickly, with a shorter period of confusion following the end of the seizure.

A complex partial seizure may arise from a simple partial seizure; that is, a seizure arising from a localized area of the brain, without loss of awareness, may evolve into a somewhat more elaborate seizure with loss of consciousness. A complex partial seizure may itself evolve into a secondary generalized tonic clonic seizure.

Secondary Generalized Tonic Clonic ("Grand Mal") Seizures

These seizures affect large portions of the brain, but start from a very localized focus in the brain. Sometimes the seizure starts slowly at its focal point, as a simple partial seizure, and as the electrical activity spreads, the symptoms also spread in a Jacksonian march (see Chapter 2). At other times, the seizure activity spreads from the focus so rapidly that even an observer can't tell that it had a focal origin. It seems as though the person has entered immediately into a generalized seizure affecting the entire body.

Eric had meningitis when he was 8 years old. He experienced several "grand mal" seizures at the time of the meningitis, but was seizure-free between the ages of 8 and 19. Then the staring-spell seizures began.

"My seizures start without any warning. All of a sudden I hear Barney Rubble talking to Fred Flintstone. *The Flintstones* was one of my favorite television cartoons when I was a child, and I really loved Barney Rubble. I can't see their cartoon figures, I can just hear them talking. Barney always says, 'Hello, neighbor.... What are you up to today, Fred?' Fred always replies, 'Hiya Barney, ol' pal.... I'm about to become rich, a millionaire. I'll be the richest guy in Bedrock.' As soon as I hear Barney Rubble, I know I'm going to have a seizure. It starts right after Fred stops talking. My co-workers say I stand motionless. I just stand in one place and stare straight ahead. It lasts about a minute. Afterwards, I blink my eyes a few times and shake my head. Then I'm usually back at work as if nothing has happened. Several times a year, though, one of these spells changes into a grand mal seizure."

In the first stage of a grand mal (generalized tonic clonic) seizure such as Eric occasionally experiences, the person gives a grunt or cry as air is suddenly forced out of the lungs, then slumps in his or her seat, or falls to the ground, unconscious and unresponsive. The body stiffens briefly and then begins to jerk. The period when the body is tense and stiff is referred to as the *tonic phase* of the seizure; the time when it is jerking is referred to as the *clonic phase*. Hence, these seizures are known as tonic clonic, and they are called *generalized* because they affect both sides of the body. The person may bite his or her tongue, and frothy, blood-tinged saliva may appear around the mouth. Breathing may be shallow; it may even stop for a few moments, which can be a terrifying experience for a family member who is present. Sometimes the skin turns a bluish or grayish color, because the breathing has been interrupted and the blood doesn't get as much oxygen as usual. After one or two minutes the jerking movements slow down and the seizure ends naturally. Bladder or bowel control may be lost as the body relaxes after the seizure. Consciousness returns slowly. The person is tired and sore, and usually doesn't feel very well. Generalized tonic clonic seizures are relatively stressful events. Some people even dislocate their shoulders or bruise themselves against floors or obstacles.

Vicky says she really doesn't know how to describe her generalized tonic clonic seizures. "Usually, the only thing I remember is waking up in an ambulance. Sometimes I don't even remember the ambulance ride. I just wake up in the hospital emergency room, feeling pretty awful. I'm sore and I usually have a headache. Sometimes I've even bitten my tongue, and that hurts a lot.

"My mother has seen many of my seizures. She says I suddenly make a funny grunting sort of sound. I then fall to the ground and go rigid as a board. I turn blue, and if I've bitten my tongue blood comes out of my mouth. I then shake all over."

Primary Generalized Seizures

Absence Seizures

Absence seizures (also called *petit mal* seizures) characteristically begin in early childhood. They may persist into the adult years, but more often they disappear in the late teenage years. A child with absence seizures will suddenly stop what he or she is doing and stare into space, completely unaware of the surroundings, and unable to respond to an anxious mother or father. The seizures start without warning and end abruptly. They last only a few seconds. The child may stop speaking in mid-sentence, staring blankly, and resume talking several seconds later without realizing that anything has happened. During the brief episode of lost awareness, there may be rapid blinking or, less commonly, slumping. Parents or teachers who are unprepared for this may lose their temper, thinking the child is being defiant or disobedient. It is important to recognize that the child is not daydreaming, and is not failing to pay attention; he or she is genuinely unaware. Quite astonishingly, these seizures can happen between four and six *hundred* times in a day. Twenty percent or more of children with absence seizures develop generalized tonic clonic seizures later in life.

"Last year my teacher kept telling me to pay more attention, and my classmates used to call me a dummy," says Malcolm. "It wasn't until this year that my seizures were diagnosed. My teacher was actually the one who suggested I go to see a doctor. Apparently, many times during the day, I would just stop and stare for five or ten seconds. My friend Colin says that sometimes my eyes would blink. All I know is that when we're reading from a book, the teacher seems to be skipping a lot. Sometimes I miss several sentences at a time."

For more about absence seizures in children, see Chapter 8.

Primary Generalized Tonic Clonic Seizures

The primary generalized tonic clonic seizure is similar to the secondary generalized tonic clonic, except that the location where the seizure originated is not apparent. In the tonic phase the person will first cry out or groan, then lose consciousness and fall, as the body grows rigid. Next, in the clonic phase, the muscles jerk and twitch. Usually these movements involve the whole body, but occasionally only the face or arms are affected. There may be shallow breathing, bluish or grayish skin, drooling and loss of bowel or bladder control. Sometimes only the clonic phase is experienced; sometimes only the tonic phase.

Myoclonic Seizures

Myoclonic seizures involve dramatic, lightning-quick jerks of a portion of the body, and can occur at any age. The whole event is over in less than a second. One rare type of myoclonic seizure is an *infantile spasm*. These tend to occur in clusters in babies, usually before six months of age. Suddenly the baby appears startled or in pain, rapidly drawing up his or her knees and raising both arms as if reaching upwards for support. If the baby is sitting upright, the head may slump forward, the arms flex and the body bend over at the waist. Infantile spasms last only a few seconds but may repeat in a series of 10 to 50 or more, many times during a day. They often occur when the baby is drowsy, just awakening or about to fall asleep.

Atonic Seizures

Atonic seizures are also referred to as *astatic* seizures or *drop attacks*. In their most minimal form, atonic seizures involve a brief nodding of the head or sagging of the body. The person's legs may sag, but people suddenly catch themselves before they fall to the ground. Someone who is seated may fall forward. In a full-blown drop attack, a standing person may dramatically crash to the floor, cracking teeth or breaking the nose. These attacks typically last one or two seconds, and the person is seldom, if ever, aware of even a brief loss of consciousness. There is no warning and after the seizure there is no confusion. People pick themselves up off the ground and immediately resume what they were doing. There is no tongue biting, no change in skin color, no loss of bowel or bladder control. Atonic seizures are frequently preceded or followed by myoclonic seizures, which may also occur during the attack. People prone to these seizures react to a number of stimuli, including flashing lights and loud sounds – anything that startles them. Atonic seizures typically begin between six months and seven years of age, but may not begin until the teenage years. It is very rare for them to begin in the adult years. They almost always occur in people who also have other seizure types.

Types of Epilepsy

People have different types of seizures, and they have different types of epilepsy. Your doctor will want to determine not only what type of seizure you have but also what type of epilepsy. This can be very important for decisions about the treatment you need. For example, someone whose epilepsy results from a head injury may experience only typical complex partial seizures, passing into a kind of dreamlike state; such a person may stare, make chewing movements, pick at clothing, mumble and do the same actions over and over again. He or she can't talk to other people while the seizure is going on. Sometimes people wander during these episodes. Since all of these spells are complex partial seizures, the person has complex partial epilepsy. Other types of epilepsy are not quite so clear-cut.

Juvenile Myoclonic Epilepsy

Juvenile myoclonic epilepsy is easily confused with other types of epilepsy. It is probably the most common form of generalized epilepsy, and it begins in adolescence. The symptoms include various types of seizures, typically occurring in the early morning. However, what is quite characteristic of juvenile myoclonic epilepsy is its response to therapy. More than 80 percent of people with this disorder can control it very well using a drug called valproic acid, or divalproex.

Benign Rolandic Epilepsy

Benign rolandic – also called benign childhood epilepsy with centro-temporal spikes – is another childhood epilepsy, with seizures generally occurring between age 3 and age 15; it is called "benign" because secondary generalized tonic clonic seizures are uncommon, and when they do occur, they tend to do so during sleep. Seizures tend to be infrequent and mild, and usually disappear by the time the person reaches 15 years of age.

Reflex Epilepsy

This type of epilepsy is characterized by seizures that are provoked by some specific mental or external stimulus. The triggering factors are multiple and may include light stimulation, video games, particular types of music, tooth brushing, hot water immersion, mental arithmetic, reading and even (for some individuals) card-playing. People with reflex epilepsy occasionally also have spontaneous seizures in the absence of a triggering factor. Of all the stimuli, a flashing light is the most common; some very photosensitive (light-sensitive) people have a seizure whenever they are exposed to such a light, or even to the flicker of light through a fence they are being driven past.

Musicogenic epilepsy (a form of reflex epilepsy)

Hans has found that every physician he meets just loves to hear a description of his seizures. They seem to fascinate everyone. "I almost had one yesterday," he says. "I was in an elevator. Just as the doors closed, I realized that the elevator music was Elton John. I quickly pushed the button for the next floor, and I was able to get off the elevator before a seizure started. Several years ago, before I realized what was causing these spells, I had a seizure every time I heard Elton John. Of course, other singers occasionally cause me to have seizures, but Elton John is by far the most successful. When I do have one of my seizures, I have a staring attack for about two minutes."

West Syndrome Epilepsy

West syndrome is a more serious type of epilepsy, characterized by infantile spasms. It tends to appear in the first year of life, and may delay mental development. The spasms are motor movements that involve the head, neck and trunk and are usually generalized. The causes of West syndrome epilepsy are multiple, and include such acquired problems as brain infections and brain tumors. The seizures tend to relent when treated with drugs such as vigabatrin or ACTH. Nevertheless, the long-term prognosis is poor and there is frequently continuing epilepsy, and cognitive problems. West syndrome may evolve into Lennox-Gastaut syndrome epilepsy. It is frequently associated with a serious brain disorder called *tuberous sclerosis* (not to be confused with tuberculosis).

Lennox-Gastaut Syndrome Epilepsy

Lennox-Gastaut syndrome epilepsy is not well defined or well understood. It is a secondary generalized form of epilepsy. It tends to appear in childhood, with many different seizure types, and is associated with mental impairment. The seizures are very difficult to control, and do not respond consistently to anticonvulsant drugs.

Landau-Kleffner Syndrome Epilepsy

Landau-Kleffner syndrome epilepsy is an unusual type that begins just as a child is learning to speak, and results in a failure of speech development. (Of course, there are many other possible causes of delayed speech development.) There may also be associated behavioral disturbances. It tends to occur primarily in boys, for unknown reasons, and generally continues through life.

Rasmussen's Encephalitis Epilepsy

Rasmussen's encephalitis epilepsy typically begins between

the ages of six and ten. It is associated with intellectual deterioration. The afflicted person has partial seizures associated with weakness on one side of the body, and the seizures do not respond well to drugs. Imaging of the brain using either an MRI or CT scan (see Chapter 4) shows that half of the brain has shrunk. The surgical removal of that half, dramatic though this may sound, is sometimes helpful in stabilizing the disorder.

Take-home points

- Types of epilepsy differ from types of seizures.
- Different types of seizures arise from different areas of the brain.
- Not all seizures involving blank spells are petit mal seizures; some are complex partial seizures, some are absence seizures.
- Not all seizures involve falling to the ground and shaking.
- There are some very unusual seizure types, involving bizarre mannerisms that may be mistaken for misbehavior or signs of mental problems.

International classification of epileptic seizures
(From the International League against Epilepsy)

I. Partial (Focal, Local) Seizures
   A. Simple Partial Seizures
      1. With motor signs
      2. With somatosensory or special sensory symptoms (peculiar feelings)
      3. With autonomic symptoms or signs
      4. With psychic symptoms
   B. Complex Partial Seizures
      1. Simple partial onset followed by impairment of consciousness
      2. With impairment of consciousness at onset
   C. Partial Seizures Evolving to Secondarily Generalized Seizures
      1. Simple partial seizures evolving to generalized seizures
      2. Complex partial seizures evolving to generalized seizures
      3. Simple partial seizures evolving to complex partial seizures evolving to generalized seizures

II. Generalized Seizures (Convulsive or Non-Convulsive)
   A. Absence Seizures
      1. Typical absences
      2. Atypical absences
   B. Myoclonic Seizures
   C. Clonic Seizures
   D. Tonic Seizures
   E. Tonic Clonic Seizures
   F. Atonic Seizures (Astatic Seizures)

III. Unclassified Epileptic Seizures

International classification of epilepsies, epileptic syndromes and related seizure disorders
(From the International League against Epilepsy)

I. Localization-related (Focal, Local, Partial)
  A. Idiopathic (Primary)
    1. Benign childhood epilepsy with centro-temporal spikes
    2. Childhood epilepsy with occipital paroxysms
    3. Primary reading epilepsy
  B. Symptomatic (Secondary)
    1. Temporal lobe epilepsies
    2. Frontal lobe epilepsies
    3. Parietal lobe epilepsies
    4. Occipital lobe epilepsies
    5. Chronic progressive epilepsia partialis continua of childhood
    6. Syndromes characterized by seizures with specific modes of precipitation
  C. Cryptogenic, Defined By:
    1. Seizure type
    2. Clinical features
    3. Etiology
    4. Anatomic localization

II. Generalized
  A. Idiopathic (Primary)
    1. Benign neonatal familial convulsions
    2. Benign neonatal convulsions
    3. Benign myoclonic epilepsy in infancy
    4. Childhood absence epilepsy (pyknolepsy)
    5. Juvenile absence epilepsy
    6. Juvenile myoclonic epilepsy (impulsive petit mal)
    7. Epilepsies with grand mal seizures (GTCS) on awakening
    8. Other generalized idiopathic epilepsies
    9. Epilepsies with seizures precipitated by specific modes of activation

B. Cryptogenic or Symptomatic
1. West's syndrome (infantile spasms, Blitz-Nick-Salaam Krämpfe)
2. Lennox-Gastaut syndrome
3. Epilepsy with myoclonic-astatic seizures
4. Epilepsy with myoclonic absences

C. Symptomatic (Secondary)
1. Non-specific cause
   a) Early myoclonic encephalopathy
   b) Early infantile epileptic encephalopathy with suppression bursts
   c) Other symptomatic generalized epilepsies
2. Specific syndromes
   a) Epileptic seizures may complicate many disease states

III. Undetermined Epilepsies
A. With Both Generalized and Focal Seizures
1. Neonatal seizures
2. Severe myoclonic epilepsy in infancy
3. Epilepsy with continuous spike waves during slow-wave sleep
4. Acquired epileptic aphasia (Landau-Kleffner syndrome)
5. Other undetermined epilepsies

IV. Special Syndromes
A. Situation-related Seizures
1. Febrile convulsions
2. Isolated seizures or isolated status epilepticus
3. Seizures occurring only when an acute or toxic event is due to factors such as alcohol, drugs, eclampsia and non-ketotic hyperglycemia

F O U R

Diagnosis

iagnosing epilepsy is not a simple matter. Epilepsy is not like diabetes, in which blood tests can measure the degree of elevation of the glucose (blood sugar) and determine the presence of the disorder; no blood test can verify whether you have epilepsy. Nor is it like diagnosing pregnancy. When a woman is pregnant, she is pregnant twenty-four hours a day, seven days a week. Epilepsy is an intermittent problem; someone may go months, or even years, between seizures, and there is no way of knowing when the next seizure will occur.

Yet a correct diagnosis is extremely important. A person diagnosed with epilepsy stands to lose certain privileges – a driver's license, for example. And a definite diagnosis usually means a daily consumption of drugs, some of which have significant side effects. Thus both the physician and the patient had better ensure that every possible effort has been made to get the diagnosis correct.

Your doctor will need answers to the following four questions:

Are the spells you are experiencing really seizures?
It's essential to differentiate your seizures from other types of spells. For example, faints, panic attacks, migraine headaches or mini-strokes can look very much like seizures. The possibility that your symptoms stem from these "seizure mimics"

Seizures or not?

Someone who has a generalized seizure is unconscious and cannot provide an accurate description of the experience. For example, Richard developed "funny spells." When asked to describe them he said, "I feel funny and I fall to the ground shaking." Everyone assumed that he had epilepsy. He was given the anticonvulsant drug phenytoin and began to experience side effects. Although Richard couldn't give a clear account of his seizures, his wife was able to tell the doctor that Richard had shaking in both arms and both legs without loss of consciousness, and returned to normal immediately after. It became clear that he did not have epilepsy, but spells that mimicked seizures. The phenytoin was stopped and his side effects ended. He was able to get his driver's license back.

---

must be eliminated before a definite diagnosis can be made (see Chapter 11).

If your spells are seizures, what type are they?
There are many types of seizure: simple partial, complex partial, absence and generalized tonic clonic (see Chapter 3). Different seizure types require different kinds of anticonvulsant medication.

What type of epilepsy is associated with the seizures you are having?
There are at least a dozen types of epilepsy (see Chapter 3), and they require different treatment and medication. Determining the type of epilepsy is crucial to selecting the correct drug.

What is the underlying cause of your seizures?
As mentioned before, seizures are a symptom, not a disease. Many brain injuries can cause seizures – head trauma, a brain tumor or a stroke, for example. It's important to establish the underlying cause of your seizures and to treat this cause.

A Three-Step Approach

In investigating these four questions, your physician needs to be organized and systematic. There are three steps to diagnosis: taking your history; examining you physically; and doing laboratory tests.

Taking your history requires a thorough interview to establish all the relevant facts. Both you and someone who has witnessed your seizures should be interviewed.

The physical examination may involve tests of your strength, sensation, coordination, eye movements and reflexes.

The third step may involve laboratory tests such as blood tests, an electroencephalogram (EEG), a computerized tomography (CT) scan, a magnetic resonance imaging (MRI) scan and possibly even a positron emission tomography (PET) scan.

Laboratory Tests

The Electroencephalogram

The EEG is a valuable diagnostic tool. An electroencephalographic reading, which is done with a machine that detects and records brain waves, provides information about the electrical functioning of the brain. However, the EEG is not by itself capable of providing a diagnosis of epilepsy. Some people with abnormal EEGs don't have seizures or epilepsy, and some people with seizures or epilepsy have normal EEGs.

The EEG was first introduced in 1924. Since then it has been widely used (and at times abused). Its usefulness and sophistication in the diagnosis of epilepsy have steadily increased.

As discussed in Chapter 2, the brain consists of billions of neurons, which generate electrical impulses that carry messages to and from all parts of the body, through the nervous system. The EEG measures this electrical activity through small metal disks, called electrodes, which are applied to the scalp, secured with a gel or paste, in key locations over the surface of the head. Electrical cables attached to the disks carry the brain's electrical impulses to the EEG machine. The impulses are displayed on a computer screen and may be printed out on paper or stored within the computer. The EEG recording is then examined for evidence of the abnormal electrical activity that is associated with seizures or epilepsy. The procedure is completely painless.

Your physician or the laboratory personnel will provide you with instructions on preparing for the EEG. You will be advised to avoid caffeine-containing drinks such as tea, coffee or cola for eight to twelve hours prior to the EEG, and asked to wash your hair thoroughly on the day of the test, so that your scalp is free of oil, hair spray, mousse and other hair preparations. You will be told to eat a regular meal or small snack two hours before the EEG, to stabilize your blood sugar level, and to take all of your normal medications, including anticonvulsant drugs. The various drugs for epilepsy normally do not interfere with the detection of epilepsy.

The technologist will measure your head to determine the correct locations for the electrodes, then scrub your scalp in these places to remove any remaining oil. At that point he or she will apply the gel, then the electrodes, to the scalp. You will be asked to perform certain actions to activate your brain waves and accentuate the electrical activity of your brain. For example, you will probably be asked to breathe rapidly and deeply for approximately three minutes (hyperventilation). This may cause some mild dizziness or tingling around your mouth; this is a normal response. Photic stimulation is also used; a bright flashing light is placed immediately in front of your closed eyes. The whole procedure of having an EEG should last 60 to 90 minutes.

The EEG has many uses in epilepsy. It can help to support the diagnosis of epilepsy, although a definite diagnosis can't be made solely on the basis of an abnormal EEG. The EEG can also help to classify the seizure type, and to locate the focus (this can be of value in selecting patients for surgery). It may be able to quantify the frequency and duration of seizures or epileptic bursts. Finally, although the EEG is not terribly valuable in determining whether a given drug is being useful – many people who experience excellent seizure control with an anticonvulsant drug show no change or improvement in their EEG – it may help your doctor decide whether anticonvulsant drugs should be stopped. This is a much-debated issue.

The EEG is a fast, inexpensive way to examine electrical activity in the brains of patients with seizures. It is extremely safe and can be repeated many times. It provides wonderful information concerning the location and nature of any abnormal electrical activities in the brain. The major disadvantage is that it records your brain for only a fixed period of time. If you have two seizures per year and the EEG records your brain-wave activity for one hour during that year, there is obviously a very high probability of missing some abnormal electrical activity. Another disadvantage is that your hair, scalp and skull are all barriers between the electrodes and your brain. These barriers tend to reduce the sensitivity of the machine's recording instruments.

In trying to understand the usefulness of EEG in epilepsy, keep a number of facts in mind. Between 15 and 20 percent of seizure patients will have a normal EEG even if it is recorded repeatedly. Approximately 2 percent of people show epileptic changes on their EEG although they have never had a seizure in their lives. In some studies, 45 percent of the first-degree relatives (parents, siblings, children) of people with primary generalized epilepsy have abnormal EEGs despite the

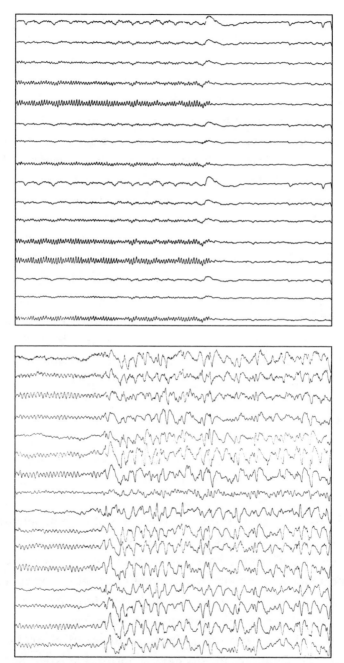

Tracings from an EEG. Top, a normal alpha rhythm (left) changes when the patient opens his eyes (right). Bottom, a normal rhythm (left) is disrupted by a generalized seizure (right).

fact that they have never had a seizure. Also, people with problems such as brain tumors or strokes may show EEG changes that look like seizures without ever having had a seizure. Medications may also influence EEG patterns. Most anticonvulsant drugs tend to slow the electrical activity in brain waves, especially if used in large doses.

Clearly, careful interpretation of the EEG is crucial. When a person is healthy, the electrical messages to and from the brain tend to produce characteristic patterns of *alpha waves* and *beta waves*. Alpha waves normally appear when the person is awake and relaxed, with eyes closed. Beta waves appear when the person is awake but is slightly tense. Certain medications, such as benzodiazepines (clobazam, clonazepam) may accentuate beta waves. The person who interprets the EEG is looking for wave patterns that are different from these normal alpha or beta waves and, in particular, for *spikes*, *sharp waves* and *spike waves*. These three abnormalities suggest the electrical activity sometimes seen in people who have various kinds of seizures or epilepsy. For instance, in complex partial seizures, sharp waves or spike waves tend to be seen from one or both temporal regions. In simple partial seizures, the EEG is sometimes normal. In absence seizures, the EEG characteristically shows a three-per-second spike-wave abnormality. All of these abnormalities may assist your doctor in determining what type of seizures you are experiencing.

Because the EEG is such an important tool in the diagnosis of epilepsy, its technology has become increasingly specialized. One simple but useful modification is the *sleep-deprived EEG*. Before this recording, the patient stays awake 24 hours. He or she is extremely tired, and may even fall asleep during the recording process. In either state – fatigued or asleep – an underlying seizure focus is more likely to be detected.

The *ambulatory EEG* is a variant of the original, stationary machine; its electrodes are connected to a portable recording device that the patient carries in a purse around his or her neck, so that diagnostic sampling can go on continuously for 24 or 48 hours. If you are having a seizure every one to two days, this ambulatory EEG will record the actual seizure. Another refinement is *video EEG monitoring*. This normally involves hospital admission so that the EEG recording can take place over a week or even longer, and be recorded on video. This allows the physician to compare the EEG abnormality to the actual symptoms. Video EEG monitoring is very useful in helping to differentiate between seizures and other spells.

Computerized Axial Tomography
The CT scan is a form of *neuro imaging*, which assesses brain structure. This scan is a form of diagnostic X-ray. A brief, carefully controlled burst of radiation is concentrated on a small part of the brain. The X-rays penetrate tissue and scan a narrow cross-section. Many scans are taken, and a computer then reconstructs them as an image on a screen. The final image, which portrays the structure of the brain, is the CT scan. It can detect sizable tumors (about as wide as a fingernail), malformations involving blood vessels, birth-related malformations, strokes, brain abscesses and bony abnormalities of the skull – any of which may be the underlying cause of seizures.

The CT scan is a very useful diagnostic tool but, like the EEG, it has limitations. It tends to miss abnormalities at the base of the brain, and it may fail to detect certain tumors. Moreover, in many cases it's unnecessary. For example, a young child with normal intelligence and a normal neurologic examination who is experiencing frequent 10-to-15-second spells of blank, unresponsive staring and eyelid fluttering does not need a CT scan. This child has absence seizures, which can be further established by the EEG, and there is no point in exposing the child to more radiation. In any case the CT scan would probably be normal. On the other hand, a young adult who has experienced three or four spells involving two minutes of blank, unresponsive staring, associated with lip-smacking, probably has complex partial seizures. Neuro imaging would definitely help the diagnostic process.

Anyone can have a CT scan. People with pieces of certain metals in them (such as shrapnel from an accident), who cannot have MRI scans, can have CT scans. However, people with kidney problems may not be able to take a contrast dye that is sometimes injected during the recording of a CT scan, to make the image easier to see. Also, some people are allergic to the dye. Having a CT scan recorded is a less claustrophobic experience than having a MRI scan recorded. A CT takes about 20 minutes to record and there are absolutely no after-effects.

Magnetic Resonance Imaging
Like the CT scan, the MRI provides structural information about the brain. MRI pictures are extremely precise. In fact, in many cases the MRI picture is so revealing that it's as if the doctor could actually see into your brain.

The MRI scanner can produce highly detailed two- or three-dimensional images. It employs a large magnet, radio waves and a computer. Unlike the CT scan, it does not use X-rays.

The way it works is quite impressive. Within the atoms that make up your brain are a series of smaller particles called protons. Under normal conditions the protons spin about randomly, but when your brain is placed near a magnet the protons line up and spin in the same direction, like so many spinning tops. If radio waves are beamed into the magnetic field, they make the protons wobble out of alignment, the way a spinning top will wobble if it is touched. When the radio wave signal is stopped, the protons will move back to their aligned position. The MRI scanner creates a magnetic field and then sends out radio waves, and a sensitive device measures the energy that the protons release as they move. This and various other measurements provide extraordinary information about the structure of the brain, which a computer converts into a high-quality picture of what the brain looks like.

Since the MRI machine employs a very strong magnet, you will be asked to remove all metallic objects before you are scanned. For instance, jewelry, glasses, clothing with zippers, even non-permanent dentures must be removed. You may even have to leave off makeup, since some cosmetics have a metallic base. You'll also have to leave your credit cards elsewhere, as the magnetism can affect their coding.

Having an MRI scan is similar to having a CT scan. For both procedures you lie on a scanning table, generally on your back. As the scan begins, the scanning table slides partly into the interior of the machine. In the case of an MRI this is a large magnet, which is like a tunnel open at both ends. During either scan it's important to stay still so that the pictures are not blurred. The procedure is painless, though some people find it claustrophobic to put their head inside the MRI scanner. Also, some MRI machines make unnervingly loud knocking and thumping sounds. However, there are no after-effects, and when the scan is finished you may readily return to your normal activities.

Although it is currently the imaging procedure of choice in epilepsy diagnosis, the MRI scan has some disadvantages. CT scan machines are still much more widely available, and much less expensive; CT scans can also be recorded more rapidly. Patients with cardiac pacemakers, surgical clips on their arteries or metallic skull plates can't have MRIs. Also, strange as it may seem, some people have metallic bodies in their eyes;

for instance, if you hit a nail, even many years ago, and a small piece of metal flew into your eye, it's probably still there. Such people can't have MRIs. If you think you may have metal in your eye, this can be checked with a regular X-ray.

Positron Emission Tomography

PET scanning is a very expensive technique, and it's available at only a small number of medical centers. While the EEG provides information about the electrical function of the brain, and neuro imaging techniques such as CT or MRI scans provide information about the structure of the brain, PET scans provide information about the chemistry of the brain, and how it may change during a seizure. A PET scan also provides useful information about brain metabolism and blood flow to various parts of the brain, as well as the action of anticonvulsant drugs. PET scanning is a very high-tech procedure and is used primarily for research. It has yet to assume a place in the day-to-day investigation and diagnosis of epilepsy.

Blood Tests

Very few neurologic conditions causing seizures can be diagnosed by means of blood tests, and their usefulness in diagnosing epilepsy is highly overrated by physicians and patients alike. Since epilepsy arises from electrical problems in the brain, it can rarely be diagnosed solely on the basis of a blood test. Nevertheless, in the interests of thoroughness, blood tests should be performed. Certain medical problems such as systemic lupus erythematosus (SLE) or acquired immune deficiency syndrome (AIDS) can cause seizures, and blood tests may be of value in detecting them. Also, if the level of sodium in a person's blood drops too low, seizures may result, and this problem will show up in routine blood tests.

Take-home points

- The history you and any witnesses give your doctor – the description of how the seizure began and what it was like – is more important in diagnosing epilepsy than any other piece of information; it is more valuable than an EEG or a CT scan.
- The EEG cannot diagnose epilepsy unless a seizure occurs during the EEG. Some people with seizures have normal EEGs; some people with abnormal EEGs don't have seizures.
- EEGs and imaging (CT, MRI scan) are complementary. EEGs provide information about the electrical functioning of the brain; imaging provides information about its anatomy.

FIVE

Drug-Based Treatment

Drugs are the most widely used treatment for epilepsy. If you have seizures, you have almost certainly been treated with drugs at some point in your life. Your experiences may have ranged from very good to terrible. There are wonderful stories of people whose seizures are perfectly controlled by medications, allowing them to participate in any activity they desire (including driving a car). On the other hand, there are horror stories of individuals who have suffered severe side effects, or have actually died, after taking an anticonvulsant.

Many drugs are presently in use against epilepsy. They work through various mechanisms, and not all of them work against all types of seizures, but when they are used correctly they are good drugs, and can be of tremendous benefit. Some of them are designed to suppress seizures by preventing the spread of abnormal electrical activity from the focus to other parts of the brain. Others are targeted toward preventing the spread of electrical excitation from one brain cell to another. To achieve this, they may act on the excitatory neurotransmitters, or they may enhance or mimic the inhibitory neurotransmitters. However, most drugs work on the surface of brain cells, to block electrical activity along the individual cells.

In this chapter, we will consider the dozen drugs that are most frequently prescribed. A table of drugs and common brand names appears at the end of the book. Terms such as *anticonvulsant, anti-epileptic* and *antiseizure* are used loosely by many medical practitioners. Doctors and patients may take these words to mean very different things. In fact, there is no such thing as a true antiepileptic drug (although physicians often use the acronym AED, even when talking to patients). None of the drugs now prescribed will prevent or cure epilepsy. If someone is in a car accident and has brain damage, that person's risk of developing epilepsy increases enormously. This post-traumatic epilepsy usually develops two years or more after the head trauma. Even if every one of the currently available "antiepileptic" drugs were used at the time of the head trauma, they would not prevent epilepsy from starting. All these drugs are able to suppress seizures, more or less effectively, in patients who have already developed epilepsy, but they do not prevent the disorder.

Beginning Drug Treatment

Your doctor will assess your condition and prescribe a drug if he or she feels it's necessary, but this is not always an easy decision. There are many opinions about what's right and what's wrong, but there are no certainties, and no doctor is right 100 percent of the time.

There are some general principles. First, "one seizure does not an epileptic make." That is, the fact that you've had a single seizure doesn't necessarily mean you should be treated with anticonvulsant drugs. It's possible that you will never have another seizure. It's the physician's job to try to determine which patients need medication to prevent further seizures, and which patients are at low risk and probably don't need anticonvulsants. (However, if a single, prolonged seizure is the result of head trauma – a fractured skull, for example – and you're having the seizure in the emergency department, you will probably, quite correctly, be treated with anticonvulsants. In those circumstances there is no doubt about the cause of the seizure, or about the seizures that will probably soon follow.)

When is it advisable to begin anticonvulsant drugs? After two seizures? After three? Most doctors start to treat with drugs after the second seizure. However, if more than a year has elapsed since the first seizure, a strong case can be made for holding off on drugs; if you are having one seizure per year, it's debatable whether you should be taking a potentially toxic drug on a daily basis. The decision must be one that both you and your physician find acceptable. If you want to operate a motor vehicle, and if that is an option where you live, you'll probably have to take anticonvulsants to decrease the chance of having a seizure at the wheel. But if you're a concert pianist, you may not want to take any drug that would slow down your hand movements on the piano keyboard, as anticonvulsants might. This is a tough decision, and all the potential risks and benefits must be taken into consideration.

How Much Is Enough?
People sometimes wonder if they should have their blood checked, to be sure the level of anticonvulsant is high enough. There is definitely no need for this. If you're not having seizures, or any toxic side effects from the medications you are taking, there is no reason to check your blood levels. The goal of your treatment is for you to be seizure-free, without side effects – not to have the anticonvulsant at a particular level in your blood.

In fact, the "normal" range of drug level in the blood may

not be normal for you. Every patient is an individual and requires individual consideration. In any case, the level of drug in your blood may not accurately reflect what is happening in your body. Various organs within the body (especially the liver) chemically alter any drug you take, in a process referred to as *metabolism*, and that process varies from person to person. When a drug is metabolized in your body it is converted to other drugs, called *metabolites*, which may be effective in eliminating seizures, or may not. Likewise, they may cause side effects, and they may not.

The main reason for checking anticonvulsant levels in the blood is to assist in medication adjustments if someone either has poorly controlled seizures, or is having side effects. There is no reason to have your blood tested routinely just because you are on anticonvulsants.

One Drug Versus Several
The ultimate objective is to have no seizures and no side effects. In aiming for this, it's best to take as few drugs as possible in as low a dosage as possible. Taking one drug is generally better than taking two or more drugs.

Chronic toxicity

Manuel is 53, and he has been on phenytoin and phenobarbital for 25 years. He has been averaging one seizure every 18 months or so for the past 5 years. He says he feels well and is having no side effects from his anticonvulsants. He denies any particular fatigue; he has always needed eight to ten hours of sleep a night, he says. He sees no reason to change his medications.

His wife disagrees, and feels that he is always tired and irritable. Finally a decision is made to taper off and stop the phenobarbital, leaving him on phenytoin alone. His seizures are no more frequent than they were when he was on both phenytoin and phenobarbital. However, he feels much better, has more energy and feels brighter about life. After being chronically tired for twenty-five years, he no longer remembered what it was like not to be tired. He assumed that this was his normal state.

Keep it simple

A hockey injury in Phil's teenage years led to a full array of seizures, including simple partial seizures, complex partial seizures and secondary generalized tonic clonic seizures. Initially he was tried on a combination of phenytoin and phenobarbital. This failed to control his seizures and gave him significant side effects. Next he was tried on phenytoin and carbamazepine. This too failed to control his seizures, and gave him significant side effects. Next he was tried on carbamazepine and valproic acid. Although this controlled his seizures, he continued to have side effects.

When the carbamazepine was stopped and he was placed on single-drug therapy with valproic acid, he experienced virtually no side effects and excellent seizure control. He has continued to do well on just valproic acid.

There are several potential problems with taking multiple drugs. The combined toxicities are likely to be greater. Also, the two drugs may interact with each other in an undesirable, competitive way, and taking two drugs tends to decrease the usefulness of measuring blood levels. In many instances, the combination delivers more toxicity than therapeutic benefit.

Taking one drug to control seizures is called *monotherapy*; taking many drugs is referred to as *polytherapy*. Monotherapy is usually better.

Taking Drugs Once or Several Times in a Day

How often should drugs be taken? There is the occasional person who actually sets an alarm clock in order not to miss a four a.m. drug dose, but this is completely unnecessary.

The frequency is best determined by the *half-life* of the drug. This is a measure of how long the drug stays in the body. Typically, a drug should be taken at intervals that match its half-life. For example, phenytoin has a half-life of twenty-four hours and thus may be taken once per day. Valproic acid has a substantially shorter half-life and must be taken several times throughout the day. When drugs are used in combinations (polytherapy) their half-lives tend to be shortened.

Storing Anticonvulsants

Store your anticonvulsant pills in a location that will help you remember to take them. It should also be a place that is dry (dampness may decrease their effectiveness) and protected from both direct sunlight and extremes of temperature. The refrigerator is *not* a good place; nor is the kitchen cupboard over the dishwasher, or the bathroom or the car glovebox. Remember that anticonvulsants are potentially lethal to children, and must be kept out of their reach.

Mistakes Happen

Don't be too worried if you accidentally miss a dose of your anticonvulsant. No one's perfect, and missed doses are extremely common. It's unlikely that missing a single dose will result in your having a seizure. However, if the drug has a very short half-life the chances are much higher.

If you realize that you've missed a single dose, take the missing medication immediately, even if your next dose is almost due. Most people tolerate a double dose without any side effects. However, if your past reactions suggest that there will be toxic side effects, divide the medication up and take it over a period of several hours.

Discontinuing Drug Treatment

At some point, your doctor may wish to stop your treatment with anticonvulsants. This too is a decision in which many variables have to be taken into consideration. If your livelihood depends on driving and you're not experiencing any side effects from your drug, you may prefer to continue, and your doctor may agree that it's better for you to do so. Alternatively, if you are having considerable side effects, both you and your doctor may be quite anxious to have you stop or change the medication. There are no hard and fast rules.

As a general policy, you should be free of seizures for a minimum of two years before any consideration is given to stopping anticonvulsants. If you have been seizure-free for four to five years, your neurologist will probably feel comfortable with slowly tapering off the drug or drugs, and after you have been seizure-free for ten to fifteen years there are many, many reasons for doing so. At that point, the risk of side effects probably outweighs any potential benefit. If you have not had a seizure for fifteen years, it is safe to assume that the original seizure focus has not been firing, because anticonvulsants are just not effective enough to have suppressed all seizures for that long.

However, your doctor will weigh factors other than the length of time you have had complete seizure control. In order to rule out other possible causes for your seizures, he or she may employ various tests, including an EEG.

The role of the EEG as a predictor for safe discontinuation of anticonvulsant drugs is controversial. It cannot be stressed too much that a normal EEG does not rule out the possibility of continuing seizures and an abnormal EEG does not reliably indicate that they will occur. Nevertheless, it's probably safe to say that, if the EEG shows an epileptic abnormality, it's not a good idea to stop the medications.

If you do go off your anticonvulsant drugs, there is always a risk that the seizures will start again. As a rule of thumb, if you have been seizure-free for two to four years, there is a 15 to 20 percent chance of seizures recurring. And if a seizure does occur, there is no guarantee that the anticonvulsant drug that worked previously will work again, though it usually does. The benefits of stopping anticonvulsant medications are obvious: side effects are eliminated. Certain side effects, such as facial hair or gum overgrowth (both from phenytoin) or substantial weight gain (from valproic acid), may require months or years before they resolve. Nonetheless, most patients feel brighter and better without their anticonvulsant medications.

Specific Drugs Used in the Treatment of Seizures

Different seizure types respond to different drugs, so it would seem reasonable that for each type of seizure there should be a "drug of choice," and that if that drug isn't successful the logical alternatives should be tried in descending order of demonstrated effectiveness. However, obtaining a clear consensus on the drug of choice for each seizure type is difficult. Medical opinion varies from continent to continent, from country to country, from neurologist to neurologist.

Nevertheless, some broad generalizations can be made. For primary generalized epilepsies, valproic acid is widely accepted as the drug of choice. Lamotrigine, benzodiazepines, and barbiturates are logical alternatives. For secondary epilepsies (simple partial seizures, complex partial seizures, secondary generalized tonic clonic seizures), either carbamazepine or phenytoin is the usual first drug of choice. After these agents, a wide variety of possibilities exists, including valproic acid, lamotrigine and topiramate.

All the same, everyone is an individual, and the drug of choice for one person is not the drug of choice for another. Here's a closer look at the dozen most-prescribed drugs.

Phenobarbital

Phenobarbital is a landmark drug. It was the first real anticonvulsant ever discovered, and it has been used more than any other drug in the treatment of epilepsy. Even today, on a world-wide basis, it is the most widely used anticonvulsant drug, particularly in developing countries. It is effective and relatively safe, and much less expensive than the newer drugs.

The cost of drugs

After 15 years of seizures, Terry had tried a wide variety of anticonvulsant drugs. He had found that a combination of valproic acid and vigabatrin gave him superb seizure control with few if any side effects. However, because he was now seizure-free, Terry lost his eligibility for government social assistance. With some difficulty he found a job, but because of his limited work history (since seizures had prevented him from working) it was a low-paying job. This created new problems: now that he was able to work, he couldn't afford the expensive medications that controlled his seizures. What could he do?

With the support of an understanding employer, Terry began to investigate cheaper drugs. He discovered that a small dose of phenobarbital worked as well as the more expensive drugs he had been using, and that he was no more tired on the phenobarbital than he had been on the combination of valproic acid and vigabatrin. He was very happy with the outcome of his research, since the phenobarbital was inexpensive and posed no financial hardship to him.

Phenobarbital belongs to a larger class of drugs referred to as barbiturates. Legend has it that the chemist who discovered these drugs named the chemical family after his girlfriend, Barbara. For a chemist, that is true love.

Phenobarbital was first employed as a sedative; it was discovered to be an anticonvulsant in Germany in 1912, when an intern physician named Hauptmann was assigned to work on a neurology ward. Many of the patients had seizures, and the seizures (as is normal) occurred more frequently at night. This would disturb the patients' sleep (as well as the sleep of Dr. Hauptmann), so he decided to give all these patients phenobarbital to help them sleep better. Quite unexpectedly, the patients began to have fewer seizures.

Phenobarbital is well absorbed; that is, if you swallow it, much of the dose is taken up into the body from the gastrointestinal tract. Its half-life ranges from 46 to 136 hours – an average of four days. This is the longest half-life of any anticonvulsant, and because of this long half-life the drug can be taken in one daily dose, rather than in divided doses, multiple times throughout the day. This simplicity is one of its great advantages. Moreover, after a person has taken a last dose, the drug tends to hang around in the bloodstream for days, even weeks.

Phenobarbital is a *broad-spectrum* anticonvulsant, active against a wide range of seizure types – unlike other anticonvulsants, which are effective against a limited range of seizures. Also, phenobarbital is used in both adults and children, including newborn babies. Its side effects include tiredness, drowsiness, dizziness, blurred vision, incoordination, skin rash and depression. The higher the dose of phenobarbital, the more likely these side effects are. Rarely, behavioral

Behavioral side effects

Sophie is in her forties and lives in a group home. She was afflicted with severe meningitis at the age of five months, which was complicated by an episode of status epilepticus (see Chapter 7). The combination of meningitis and status epilepticus left her mentally handicapped.

Sophie's aging parents and the group home directors are happy with her seizure control: she has a generalized tonic clonic seizure about once every two years, and staring spells a couple of times per month, but no one is much concerned about the latter. However, there is concern about her behavior, which is sometimes aggressive and violent. She will throw things across the room, or strike herself in the head with her own hands. Sophie has been on phenytoin and phenobarbital for at least 20 years. She has probably been on them for longer than that, but the records have been lost.

The phenobarbital was tapered off over a period of several months. About two months after it was stopped, people at the group home noticed a dramatic change in Sophie's behavior. The violent outbursts stopped. She became much happier and more contented. Although she was receiving phenytoin alone, her seizure frequency didn't change.

Over the ensuing year, the phenytoin was gradually replaced by carbamazepine. Although there was a further improvement in her behavior, her seizures worsened slightly. With an increasing dose of carbamazepine, however, her seizures almost completely disappeared. She continues to do well.

side effects are produced. Paradoxically, in younger children phenobarbital can produce agitation and excitability.

When taken over a long period of time, phenobarbital can produce impaired concentration and thinking, and possibly behavioral disturbances in some individuals. Long-term use can also affect vitamin D and calcium chemistry within the body, producing or aggravating underlying osteoporosis; this is most relevant for women who are already susceptible to bone thinning. Long-term use can also affect folic acid chemistry, occasionally causing mild anemia. Finally, if phenobarbital is abruptly stopped after long-term administration, there may be withdrawal symptoms, including seizures.

Primidone

Like phenobarbital, primidone has been around for a very long time. In fact, the two drugs are closely related and from a chemical perspective the primidone molecule is quite similar to the phenobarbital molecule. However, these are not identical drugs. Primidone itself has anticonvulsant activity, and it is converted by the body to phenobarbital and to another chemical called phenylethylmalonamide (PEMA). Both phenobarbital and PEMA also have anticonvulsant activity, although PEMA appears to be a relatively weak anticonvulsant. Thus taking primidone is like taking a mixture of primidone, phenobarbital and PEMA. Some physicians argue that a complementary effect is created by using phenobarbital and primidone together. Others disagree, and the bulk of opinion suggests that, because of their combined toxicity, the risks of taking both together outweigh any benefits.

Like phenobarbital, primidone works against a wide range of seizure types. However, it tends to work best against tonic clonic seizures and partial seizures. It also has some use against myoclonic seizures.

The side effects of primidone are similar to those of phenobarbital, except that primidone is even less well tolerated. The side effects of large doses include drowsiness, fatigue, dizziness, incoordination and blurred vision; vitamin D, calcium and folic acid depletion; diminished libido and sexual dysfunction; and skin rash. The drug can also cause problems with concentration.

Phenytoin

Phenytoin has a long history. It was first evaluated as a sleeping pill, but was found to have anticonvulsant effects as well; these effects were investigated in the mid-1930s by two researchers in the United States, who tested the drug's anti-seizure properties on cats. Within several months it was being used by human beings. (In those days, there were no laws requiring protracted clinical trials.)

Phenytoin does not work on all seizure types. It tends to work better on secondary epilepsies. Thus it works best for tonic clonic seizures and partial seizures. It is not typically used for primary generalized epilepsies. It can be given intravenously, and is often used in emergencies, for uncontrolled seizures.

When phenytoin is first started, or when the dose is increased too fast, side effects may include dizziness, incoordination, imbalance, slurred speech, tremor, confusion and impaired concentration. Also, when the person looks towards the right or left, the eyes may show a coarse jerking movement called *nystagmus*. If these side effects don't settle down in several days, they usually subside with a reduction in dose.

More noteworthy are the chronic side effects associated with phenytoin. The most common ones are overgrowth of the gums (*gingival hyperplasia*), facial hair in women (*hirsutism*) and acne. Not surprisingly, these side effects are not appreciated by patients.

Physical side effects of phenytoin

Elena has had spells for two years, in the form of blank, unresponsive staring episodes. Once or twice these episodes, which were apparently caused by a bicycle accident seven years ago, have progressed to a full generalized tonic clonic seizure. At first Elena was reluctant to use any medications, but she wanted to get her driver's license back, and agreed to try phenytoin. Within eight months she had become quite depressed. She had developed significant acne and facial hair, and her gums were enlarged and growing down over her teeth. She didn't know what was causing these cosmetic changes, and was despondent about them. When she learned that these were side effects of phenytoin, she became quite bitter.

Sophie's physician suggested a switch to carbamazepine. Within fourteen months the cosmetic side effects had almost entirely resolved. She still has a single complex partial seizure about once every six months, but she refuses to try changing her anticonvulsant drug because of her bad experience with phenytoin.

This medication need be taken only once a day, and is usually taken at bedtime; in fact, all three or four capsules of the average dose can be taken together at bedtime. However, getting the dosage right can be tricky. Unlike the other anticonvulsants, phenytoin has a property called *nonlinear kinetics*. What this means is that doubling the oral dose may more than double the drug's concentration in the blood. Sometimes a very minor increase in the oral dose can lead to a dramatic increase in the level of the drug in the blood, and thus to toxicity. Adjusting the dose to suit the patient can present a challenge.

Phenytoin interacts with a fairly large number of other drugs. It may reduce the effectiveness of warfarin (a blood thinner), oral contraceptives, prednisone (an anti-inflammatory steroid), furosemide (a diuretic), carbamazepine and lamotrigine. When you are starting other new drugs, or stopping old ones, your doctor must always consider the wide range of drug interactions involving phenytoin.

Loss of balance and coordination

Frank is 24. About 18 months ago he had a single generalized tonic clonic seizure. A CT scan and EEG at that time were normal, and it was decided not to treat him with anticonvulsants. About four months later he had two generalized seizures, and he was put on phenytoin at 300 mg once a day.

At that dosage Frank continued to have seizures, but when the dose was increased to 400 mg a day the seizures stopped. However, within six weeks of going on the increased dosage Frank began to experience marked difficulties with balance and coordination. He began to stagger and to feel unwell. When his dose was dropped back to 300 mg the seizures recurred; when it was increased back to 400 mg the toxicity recurred. He and his doctor agreed to try splitting the difference, and Frank started on 350 mg a day. It worked extremely well; Frank now has excellent seizure control with no side effects.

Ethosuximide

When phenytoin was first discovered to be an anticonvulsant, any chemical or molecule that even vaguely resembled it was evaluated as a potential drug for epilepsy. Ethosuximide is one of those drugs. It bears a certain resemblance to phenytoin, but it's only effective against absence seizures. It doesn't work on any of the secondary epilepsies, or against simple partial or complex partial seizures, and it has no effect on epilepsies that begin in adulthood.

The most common side effects are related to high doses. They include drowsiness, fatigue, headaches, hiccups and nausea. Allergic side effects are quite rare with this medication, but they may include skin rash, and also bone marrow depression. (The bone marrow stops producing red blood cells, white blood cells and platelets. This may lead to fatigue, infections and bleeding problems.) There are no other significant long-term side effects.

Interactions between ethosuximide and other drugs are uncommon and minor, and this drug has no interaction with oral contraceptives.

Carbamazepine

Like phenytoin, carbamazepine is probably one of the most widely used anticonvulsants. It too was discovered more by accident than by design. It was initially used as an antidepressant, but it soon became clear that the drug's anticonvulsant properties were much more marked, and it is now used mainly for these properties.

Carbamazepine has been around for approximately 40 years. Its properties are well understood and most physicians are quite comfortable prescribing it. Interestingly, many patients who have poor seizure control on phenytoin alone, or carbamazepine alone, have superb seizure control when the two agents are used together. However, there are also many people whose seizures respond well to carbamazepine but not to phenytoin, and vice versa.

Like phenytoin, carbamazepine is used primarily for secondary epilepsies. Its main use is in the treatment of tonic clonic seizures, complex partial seizures and simple partial seizures. It's probably the current drug of choice for the initial treatment of complex partial seizures. It is of no value against absence seizures.

A number of dose-related side effects occur, including double vision, headaches, dizziness, incoordination, drowsiness and tiredness. In fact, when carbamazepine is started, many patients experience double vision and incoordination in the first four to six weeks.

Carbamazepine is generally well tolerated when used chronically. A rare side effect that is sometimes observed, particularly in the elderly, is cardiac arrhythmia – a disturbance in the heart's electrical conduction – so carbamazepine should probably be used with caution in elderly people with heart conduction problems. Like other traditional anticonvulsants, carbamazepine can influence vitamin D and calcium metabolism.

Auras

Phyllis is 27. From age 12 to 22 she had severe migraine headaches, invariably preceded by an aura in the form of bright flashing lights in her visual field. The aura was followed by a severe pounding headache at the back of her head, associated with nausea, vomiting and sensitivity to light. She has a strong family history of migraine.

Over the past five years her migraines have changed. Recently, there were two occasions when she had the aura of flashing lights, but then a generalized tonic clonic seizure occurred. A co-worker suggested that Phyllis was having seizures, but she firmly believed that these were simply a variant of her migraine headache problem. Although she didn't think it necessary, at the urging of her friends she sought medical advice.

Phyllis's neurologic examination was normal. A CT scan of her head was normal, but an EEG showed generalized paroxysmal discharges. She was diagnosed as having migraine with seizures, and the seizures responded well to a small dose of carbamazepine.

Carbamazepine interacts with a number of other drugs. Oddly, the drug with which it interacts most is itself. This is a phenomenon referred to as *auto induction*. Sometimes, after people have spent several weeks or several months on carbamazepine, the dose has to be increased to maintain satisfactory seizure control. This is because carbamazepine actually enhances the body's capacity to deal with it.

Valproic Acid (Divalproex)

Valproic acid is structurally unique, and its properties and toxicities are different from those of other anticonvulsants. Valproic acid can cause weight gain, hair loss and tremor, but generally with less confusion and fatigue than are associated with the other drugs. Also, valproic acid is a broad-spectrum anticonvulsant. It works against virtually all seizure types: primary generalized seizures such as absence seizures, myoclonic seizures, tonic and atonic seizures, as well as secondary seizures such as secondary generalized tonic clonic seizures, complex partial

Valproic acid

Odette is 21, and ever since she was 17 she has had generalized tonic clonic seizures, always in the early morning hours. She was treated with carbamazepine and phenytoin in the past but these proved to be ineffective. When she is treated with valproic acid she improves dramatically and her seizures stop. She is diagnosed with juvenile myoclonic epilepsy.

On the phenytoin and carbamazepine she experienced side effects such as fatigue and incoordination. Now the valproic acid presents her with a new range of side effects. First she gains weight; she puts on 30 pounds (almost 15 kilos). Then her hair begins to fall out. When her physicians are reluctant to stop the valproic acid, she persists with the drug and her hair grows back in (slightly curlier). Next she experiences a tremor, which worries her – she is afraid her seizures are worsening. However, she is reassured by her physicians that this is yet another side effect of the valproic acid, and in fact it disappears when the dose is reduced. Odette finally resigns herself to the weight gain, because controlling her seizures is more important to her.

seizures and simple partial seizures. There is virtually no seizure type that is not suppressed to some degree by this drug.

Valproic acid has a number of side effects that distinguish it from the other drugs. Nausea and gastrointestinal upset are relatively common. Many people complain about having "the burps" on this drug, or say that their stomachs "just don't feel right." This discomfort can be minimized by taking the drug on a full stomach, dividing the dose into installments or using an enteric-coated version. Many people gain unwanted weight on this drug. Various studies have suggested that one in five people on valproic acid has weight gain, which may run from several pounds to 60 pounds (almost 30 kilos). A small percentage of people also experience hair loss, from mild thinning to substantial loss. This side effect is reversible. The hair will regrow, although sometimes with a greater amount of curl, after the drug is discontinued. The hair loss can be intermittent and recurrent, and can occur anytime while someone is on the drug.

In addition to these unusual toxicities, valproic acid, like all other anticonvulsants, has side effects that are seen when the drug is initiated or when the doses are increased. The most characteristic dose-related side effect is tremor. If you are prescribed valproic acid at a dose exceeding 1,750 mg per day, you may develop a fine hand tremor. Many patients find it upsetting to have "the shakes" and misinterpret it as a worsening of their seizures, but it's simply a side effect of the drug. It's not related to the underlying seizure disorder.

Independent of dose are the "idiosyncratic" side effects, which are unpredictable and can occur in any patient, regardless of dose. For example, an inflammation of the pancreas, called pancreatitis, has been seen, and a considerable degree of attention has been given over the years to liver problems induced by valproic acid. In children under the age of two who are receiving valproic acid in conjunction with other anticonvulsant drugs, the incidence of fatal liver failure is approximately one in 500; the risk declines with age. In adults receiving only valproic acid, the risk of severe, potentially life-threatening liver toxicity is approximately one in 45,000. Thus this drug should not be used by people who have pre-existing hepatitis or other liver disease.

Clonazepam

This drug, together with nitrazepam and diazepam, belongs to a larger family of drugs called 1, 4-benzodiazepines. Many drugs within this family are used as sleeping agents or to reduce anxiety. They are sometimes used to prevent alcoholics in withdrawal from experiencing the "DTs" (delirium tremens).

Benzodiazepines have excellent anticonvulsant properties, and are sometimes given intravenously as emergency drugs to stop seizures during status epilepticus. The main problem in using them as anticonvulsants is that people tend to develop a tolerance for their anticonvulsant effects; the drug is helpful for several weeks and then stops working. This problem of tolerance limits the use of 1,4-benzodiazepines for the treatment of epilepsy, but it in no way diminishes their utility in emergency situations.

Most 1,4-benzodiazepines have been tried in pill form for the treatment of seizures at one time or another. Nitrazepam and clonazepam have enjoyed more widespread use for epilepsy. There are some problems with sedation and tiredness from these two drugs; indeed, they are also used as sleeping pills. Drooling can be another side effect, especially with nitrazepam.

Ultimately, among the 1,4-benzodiazepines, clonazepam has probably enjoyed the greatest success as an orally administered anticonvulsant. It is most frequently used as add-on or *adjunctive* therapy, along with another drug, in the treatment of either primarily generalized or secondary seizures. Like valproic acid, clonazepam works against a wide spectrum of seizure types. It even works against the difficult-to-control seizures of Lennox-Gastaut syndrome.

In general, clonazepam is a rather safe drug. In addition to drowsiness, dose-related side effects may include some incoordination. Very rarely, clonazepam actually produces an increase in seizures. The combination of valproic acid and clonazepam can lead to a worsening of seizures, especially in the form of uncontrolled absence seizures. When used chronically, clonazepam can produce sedation, swelling of the legs and some memory difficulties.

Finally, a major drawback with clonazepam is the rapid development of tolerance in approximately 50 percent of patients. The drug may simply stop working.

Clobazam

Clobazam is a 1,5-benzodiazepine. This subtle chemical distinction (which refers to the location of nitrogen atoms in the drug molecule) means fewer problems with development of

---

How do seizures relate to the menstrual cycle?

Some women note a definite relationship between their menstrual cycle and their susceptibility to seizures, a phenomenon referred to as *catamenial epilepsy*. As a general rule, the hormone estrogen tends to be *proconvulsant* (making seizures more likely) while the hormone progesterone tends to be anticonvulsant. At different times throughout the menstrual cycle, the balance between these two hormones varies. When the balance is tipped in favor of estrogen, seizures are more likely to occur. Accordingly, in women with the catamenial predilection, the peak times for seizures are approximately five days prior to the onset of menstrual bleeding and at the time of ovulation. This tendency occurs in only 12 to 15 percent of women with epilepsy, and they may also have seizures at other times during their menstrual cycle.

---

tolerance to the anticonvulsant action than there are with clonazepam. For this reason, clobazam is probably the benzodiazepine of choice in the treatment of seizures at the present time.

It is effective against all seizure types, and as add-on therapy in the treatment of primary generalized and partial seizure disorders, including Lennox-Gastaut syndrome. In addition, clobazam can be used intermittently to treat seizures associated with the menstrual cycle. This is called *pulse therapy*. Many women experience seizures five days before the onset of menstrual bleeding. If clobazam is started just prior to the anticipated onset of seizures, it may suppress seizures for seven to ten days.

As with the 1,4-benzodiazepines, clobazam is well tolerated and its side effects are usually mild. The dose-related side effects include drowsiness, dizziness, fatigue, incoordination and occasionally excess salivation. Sudden stopping of clobazam can precipitate seizures.

Vigabatrin

The appearance of vigabatrin heralded a new era of anticonvulsant drugs in the 1980s (in Europe) and the 1990s (in Canada). As of this writing, vigabatrin has not been approved in the United States. Unlike the earlier anticonvulsants, vigabatrin was not stumbled upon by accident; it was thought out and designed.

The evolution of this drug took a long time. Early during the course of its development, it was noted that dogs developed vacuoles (tiny holes) in the white matter of their brains when receiving vigabatrin. This led to concerns that delayed the development of vigabatrin as an anticonvulsant drug. (Some side effects are species-specific. Epilepsy is quite common in dogs, and veterinarians typically use phenobarbital as the drug of choice. Many of the anticonvulsants widely used in humans are toxic for dogs. Thus, using dogs to assess toxicity for people is not ideal.) Vigabatrin continued to be developed in Europe, and eventually it was shown that the toxicity with vacuoles didn't occur in humans. Vigabatrin is now recognized as a very potent and effective anticonvulsant.

Typically, it is started as add-on therapy to treat either simple partial or complex partial seizures, with or without secondary generalization to tonic clonic convulsions. Vigabatrin works very well for the secondary or acquired epilepsies, but does not work for primary generalized epilepsies. In fact, vigabatrin can dramatically worsen absence-type epilepsy. If your seizures have been suppressed by vigabatrin used as an add-on, your doctor may want to discontinue the first drug and leave you on vigabatrin alone.

Unfortunately, between 2 and 4 percent of people on vigabatrin experience psychosis or severe depression, and it should not be used by anyone who has a history of psychiatric disorders, although these problems tend to reverse once the vigabatrin is stopped. Recently it has also been recognized that vigabatrin can produce visual-field distortions. Finally, for a small proportion of people vigabatrin's anticonvulsant effects quit working after a while; these people have developed a tolerance.

Like every anticonvulsant, vigabatrin has dose-related side effects. These include fatigue, drowsiness, headache and incoordination. With chronic use, vigabatrin has been implicated in weight gain.

Gabapentin

Like vigabatrin, gabapentin was designed and created, not discovered accidentally. A growing body of evidence suggests that, beyond its anticonvulsant properties, it may be useful in the treatment of pain disorders, especially the neuralgias associated with diabetes and shingles.

As an anticonvulsant, gabapentin is used as add-on therapy for partial and secondary generalized seizures. It is of no benefit in the treatment of primary generalized epilepsies such as absence epilepsy. Like vigabatrin, it has a narrow spectrum of indication; that is, it can only be used for certain types of seizures.

For people who have very severe epilepsy, gabapentin is probably not as potent as some of the other newer anticonvulsants, such as vigabatrin, lamotrigine or topiramate.

Drugs upon drugs

Marigold is 72. Last year she had a small stroke that left her with minimal weakness on the left side of her body, and now, as a result, she has developed simple partial seizures, and simple partial seizures spreading into generalized tonic clonic seizures. Drug treatment presents problems because she is on multiple other medications. She takes warfarin, since she has a mechanical heart-valve replacement, and a variety of other medications for her heart and for high blood pressure. Routine blood work has shown some minimal abnormalities in her liver function tests.

Phenytoin interacts badly with Marigold's other medications, and carbamazepine makes her violently dizzy. When her physician suggested gabapentin, she was reluctant, because a neighbor had used gabapentin for seizures and had found it relatively ineffective. However, when Marigold tried it she was very pleased. It controlled her seizures and she had no side effects.

However, gabapentin's claim to fame is based on its low toxicity and lack of drug interactions. It is extremely useful for seizures in elderly people, who are more susceptible to toxicity. Dose-related side effects include drowsiness, dizziness, fatigue and incoordination, but these tend to be mild and uncommon. Severe allergic reactions are rare. No chronic side effects have been described to date.

Lamotrigine

Lamotrigine is an extremely effective new anticonvulsant. It too is a product of drug design; however, the chemists who created it were testing a theory that turned out to be wrong. Lamotrigine works well at suppressing seizures, but the mechanism that makes it effective is not the one its designers were investigating. So its discovery was deliberate – but also accidental.

Like valproic acid and the benzodiazepines, lamotrigine works against virtually all seizure types. It's used as add-on treatment for primary generalized seizures (primary generalized tonic clonic, myoclonic, absence, atonic, tonic) and for partial seizures (simple partial seizures, complex partial seizures, secondary generalized tonic clonic seizures). It can also be used alone. It has some effectiveness against Lennox-Gastaut syndrome epilepsy.

The only major drawback is that lamotrigine has been implicated in causing a rash. Five to 10 percent of people develop this rash during the first six weeks of therapy, and 1 to 2 percent of people, often children, develop a severe form of rash that can be life-threatening. The chance of the rash is increased if the person is also on valproic acid.

Aside from this rash, the major dose-related effects are headache, double vision, insomnia and tiredness, dizziness and incoordination.

Topiramate

Topiramate is another recent addition to the anticonvulsant selection. It has a chemical structure like no other anticonvulsant; in fact, it is derived from a sugar called fructose, although it doesn't taste sweet. It works against a wide range of seizure types. It's used as add-on therapy to treat partial and secondary generalized seizures, and it works well against simple partial, complex partial and secondary generalized tonic clonic seizures. It also appears to be useful against various types of primary generalized seizures.

Topiramate has a number of distinctive side effects. Some people experience cognitive difficulties on this drug; they say that they have trouble thinking, that their thoughts are befuddled and confused. This is more likely to occur if the drug is started at high doses. As well, about 10 percent of people experience weight *loss*. This can be quite dramatic; apparently they have no appetite and just forget to eat. Finally, about 1.5 percent of people on vigabatrin develop kidney stones.

Other Agents

Tiagabine is a new antiseizure drug, effective against simple partial seizures, complex partial seizures and secondary generalized seizures. Adverse effects may include dizziness, drowsiness, headaches and tremor.

Felbamate is a somewhat controversial anticonvulsant, active against a wide range of seizure types, including absence seizures, and partial seizures with or without secondary spread to generalized seizures. Most significantly, felbamate shows an excellent ability to suppress the seizures associated with Lennox-Gastaut syndrome, a form of epilepsy that is very difficult to control. Regrettably, felbamate is associated with significant toxicity. Eight cases of liver failure and 21 cases of bone marrow failure have been reported in association with its use. A number of people have died as a result of these toxicities. Felbamate is available in the U.S. but has not been licensed for use in Canada.

Oxcarbazepine is very similar to carbamazepine. Their chemical structures are closely related and they work against the same seizure types. The main difference is that oxcarbazepine has less toxicity. Double vision and dizziness are slightly less with oxcarbazepine. Oxcarbazepine is also less likely to produce allergic skin rashes.

Levetiracetam is a new antiseizure drug effective against simple partial seizures, complex partial seizures and secondary generalized seizures. Adverse effects may include tiredness or dizziness. It has no recognized interactions with other antiseizure drugs.

Take-home points

- The decision to start drug treatment can be a difficult one. Most doctors do not prescribe anticonvulsants after a single seizure.
- Stopping anticonvulsants can occasionally be tricky, but most doctors will consider having you do so when you have been seizure-free for more than two years.
- Taking one drug to suppress seizures is generally better than taking two drugs.
- There are many anticonvulsants. Some are useful for only certain types of seizures, and all of them have potential side effects, some serious.

S I X

Surgical Treatment

Surgical treatment for epilepsy is usually reserved for patients who have partial seizures that are *refractory* – that is, that persist as a problem despite the use of optimal drugs and medical management. Surgery is a major undertaking. It can change a person's life; infrequently, it can be dangerous. Only about 15 percent of those with refractory partial seizures are treated surgically, though in recent years there has been a trend to operate on such people at younger and younger ages. Before the final decision to operate is made, extensive clinical data and laboratory investigations are required. You, as the patient (or parent of the patient), must be given an honest and realistic explanation of what is going to happen. What are the risks? What is the likelihood of success?

A surgical approach may be considered for adults or children who have chronic, refractory, partial or secondary generalized seizures. The surgical removal of a seizure focus is considered only when the origin of all, or at least almost all, seizures can be localized to one area of the brain, and when that region can be removed without significant harm to the patient.

Refractory (or *intractable*) seizures may be defined in different ways; there is no standard number that defines an intractable condition. Many factors play a role, including the length of the seizures and their severity, and whether the person is falling and getting hurt, and whether quality of life is seriously affected by the seizures. Social difficulties caused by the seizures will also be taken into consideration.

Finally, the decision to have seizure surgery is agreed on by both the patient (who must want to have the surgery) and the physician or surgeon (who must be willing to perform it). The patient (or a family member who bears this responsibility) must have a clear understanding of all the implications of the decision. Brain surgery must not be entered into lightly. On the other hand, when seizure surgery is successful, it has the capacity to dramatically improve the person's quality of life. Remember, though, that the purpose of epilepsy surgery is to make an unmanageable problem manageable, with or without anticonvulsants. Surgery should not be seen as an alternative to medication.

If a decision to have surgery is made, the first step is electroencephalography, in many cases including EEG video telemetry, to localize the point of seizure onset. Next, an MRI scan is performed; this is now mandatory for everyone having seizure surgery, to spot problems such as benign brain tumors, blood vessel abnormalities and brain scarring from seizures. Finally, there must be a careful neuropsychological assessment to determine, among other things, where the speech center is located in this particular person's brain, and what problems, such as decreased memory, may occur as a result of the surgery.

Seizure surgery is normally performed in hospitals or centers that specialize in the procedure, and the specifics of the surgical approach will not be the same in all hospitals, or for all patients and all seizure types. The hospital stay may be a long one. During the actual procedure, the patient is anesthetized and a network of EEG electrodes may be placed directly on the surface of the brain. The patient then returns to his or her room for monitoring. Any seizures are carefully recorded, perhaps over days or weeks. Once the seizure focus has been identified, the patient is taken back to the operating room to have the focus removed. Frequently the patient is awakened during the procedure, to ensure that no vital part of the brain (such as the part responsible for speech) is removed during the removal of the seizure focus. These procedures are usually successful, but there is no guarantee that the seizures will not return.

Types of Surgery

Temporal Lobectomy

Anterior temporal lobectomy is by far the most common surgical procedure for epilepsy, because the two temporal lobes are areas where seizures – especially complex partial seizures – frequently originate. Usually the anterior (front) three to four centimeters (roughly one and a half inches) are removed from whichever temporal lobe contains the seizure focus. The procedure tends to be slightly more successful if it is done in the non-dominant half of the patient's brain, because the dominant hemisphere is the side in which the ability to speak is located; the non-dominant hemisphere doesn't have the same commitment to speech. (In a right-handed person the left hemisphere is dominant; in left-handed people, either hemisphere could be dominant.) It is therefore essential to identify the dominant hemisphere prior to surgery. Removing the temporal lobe, be it dominant or non-dominant, will of course have certain side effects; the most common are decreases in the visual field, and possibly some memory impairment.

When Greg's seizures began, his friends thought he'd gone crazy. He'd stop and stare off into the distance with a weird look on his face. Although both Greg and his wife passionately argued that he was "definitely not crazy," his family physician, at a loss to know what to do, sent him to a psychiatrist. He was diagnosed as depressed and started on antidepressant drugs, but his spells only became more intense, and longer in duration. His medication dosage was then increased; his spells worsened. He became genuinely depressed at this time.

Hockey was one of the few things that gave Greg any pleasure in life, and he began attending more and more games, as a spectator. (He was no longer able to play because of his spells and the incoordination caused by his medications.) He had one of his spells at a hockey game, and an orthopedic surgeon sitting beside him observed what was happening. When it was over, he told Greg that it had looked to him like a temporal lobe seizure. The orthopedic surgeon arranged for Greg to see a neurologist.

Greg's physical examination was normal but his EEG demonstrated a strongly active seizure focus in the right temporal lobe of the brain, probably caused by a hockey injury 15 years earlier. He was initially treated with high doses of carbamazepine. This failed to control his seizures and over the next 6 years he tried other drugs, including phenytoin, primidone, valproic acid, clobazam, vigabatrin, gabapentin and lamotrigine. Some agents partially suppressed his seizures but most caused side effects.

Finally a surgical procedure was performed. Greg had a right anterior temporal lobectomy. He immediately became seizure-free. He was placed on carbamazepine for one year but eventually even this was stopped. He was seizure-free for two and a half years. Eventually his seizures returned, but they were now well controlled with carbamazepine, and Greg is once again seizure-free.

Portion of Brain Removed in an Anterior Temporal Lobectomy

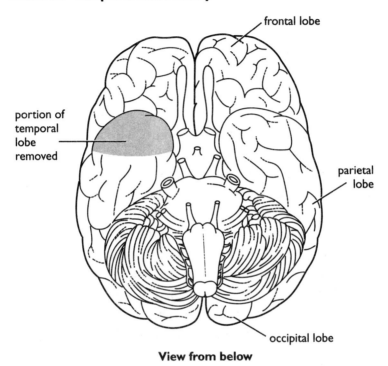

frontal lobe

portion of temporal lobe removed

parietal lobe

occipital lobe

View from below

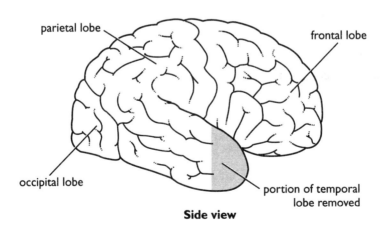

parietal lobe

frontal lobe

occipital lobe

portion of temporal lobe removed

Side view

A variant of the temporal lobectomy is a *selective amygdalo-hippocampectomy*. This procedure involves the removal of brain parts called the amygdala and the hippocampus; it's a smaller version of the temporal lobectomy described above. This is not possible for all patients, but it entails less risk of visual field defects, speech abnormalities and memory impairment. Moreover, if necessary the procedure can be extended to more comprehensive surgery, such as temporal lobectomy.

Not all complex partial seizures arise from the temporal lobe. There are also *extra-temporal* complex partial seizures. The small area of brain associated with these can sometimes be identified and successfully removed.

Bob had had seizures for 20 years when his neurologist decided that he was a suitable candidate for surgery. His seizures had always been very similar in nature, drugs had been ineffective and multiple EEGs had demonstrated a right-hemisphere seizure focus in the temporal lobe. Bob underwent an anterior right temporal lobectomy.

Since the surgery, he has been on one-drug therapy with carbamazepine. He has about one complex partial seizure per year. He is disappointed that he still can't have a driver's license but, since his seizure frequency has dropped from more than 70 per year to one, he is generally pleased. However, he is quick to point out that he has not been cured. His wife also has mixed feelings; she says that he's become different – "not the man I married." She finds it difficult to define exactly how Bob is different. His memory is worse, she says, and before the surgery he always found television cartoons silly and insipid (as did she). Now he finds them hilariously funny. She doesn't know if this has arisen directly from surgery ("did they cut out the brain center that mercifully let him hate cartoons?") or indirectly ("has he had a change in philosophy of life following this major surgery?")

Temporal lobectomy is usually successful. Sixty-five to 70 percent of those who undergo it become seizure-free; another 20 to 25 percent have a significant reduction in seizures. (These figures apply to anterior temporal lobectomy. Extratemporal surgery, to remove small areas not in the lobe, is less satisfactory, with only 30 to 50 percent of patients becoming seizure-free.)

Hemispherectomy

Hemispherectomy is considered only for children, usually under age 12, with severe, intractable seizures arising from an injury isolated to one half of the brain. This usually results from birth-related malformations, an unusual disorder called Rasmussen's encephalitis (see Chapter 3) or an uncommon blood-vessel abnormality of the brain called Sturge-Weber syndrome. In this procedure, the functional components of one of the brain's hemispheres are surgically removed. Although this is a drastic step, children who undergo the procedure show an amazing capacity to bounce back and adjust. They recover quite well. With functional hemispherectomy, 75 to 80 percent of patients become seizure-free. Their behavior is also frequently improved. Moreover, they retain their ability to walk.

Corpus Callosotomy

The *corpus callosum* is a band of tissue located between the two brain hemispheres. By conducting electricity it permits the two hemispheres to "talk to each other." When someone has severe drop attacks – seizures in which he or she collapses to the ground – the corpus callosum can be cut to prevent the seizures from spreading from one hemisphere to the other. Typically only the front two-thirds of the corpus callosum is cut at first. If necessary, this procedure can later be extended to a complete *callosotomy*. Corpus callosotomy significantly reduces drop attacks in 50 to 75 percent of patients.

Risks and Benefits

The overall risk of severe complications from epilepsy surgery is approximately one percent. The nature and severity of these complications depend on the type and extent of the surgical procedure. For example, some people are depressed for several months following surgery. Very rarely, a left temporal lobectomy produces an inability to speak. Rarely, psychosis develops in years following temporal lobectomy.

All the same, seizure surgery can be a dramatic and effective way of curing a seizure disorder in someone who has suffered from seizures and drug toxicities for years.

Vagal Stimulation

In recent years, a very new type of surgical therapy for epilepsy has emerged, called *vagal stimulation*. A vagal stimulator is a small pulse generator that is placed underneath the skin, at the front of the patient's chest. A wire is then tunneled upwards, under the skin, into the neck. Within the neck, the wire is curled around the *vagus* nerve. When the device fires, it stimulates the vagus nerve, which sends an electrical signal up to the brain. This changes the concentrations of several chemicals in the brain, achieving the goal of seizure suppression. Typically, the pulse generator is set to fire at fixed intervals throughout the day. If the person has an aura and feels a seizure about to come on, he or she can manually trigger the vagal stimulator and possibly abort the seizure.

Vagal stimulators are rapidly gaining popularity. They seem to work best for people who have complex partial seizures with seizure foci in both temporal lobes. These people are not candidates for routine seizure surgery, because it's not possible to cut out both temporal lobes, so – if they fail to respond to anticonvulsants – the vagal stimulator may be of great value in helping them suppress seizures. It's generally pain-free and easy to use. Side effects may include sore throat, hoarseness, shortness of breath and pain at the site of stimulation. Vagal stimulators cost thousands of dollars and are not usually covered by health insurance.

Take-home points

- Seizure surgery should be considered for people who, despite careful medical management, continue to have intractable seizures.
- Anterior temporal lobectomy, for the treatment of complex partial seizures, is the most widely used seizure surgery.
- Rarely, seizure surgery can be as drastic as removal of half the brain (hemispherectomy); this is done only for young children, who generally recover extremely well.
- Vagal stimulation is an emerging form of seizure surgery.

Medical Emergencies

Seizures are sudden, dramatic events, and seizure disorders often lead to medical emergencies.

Sometimes, the emergency is not related directly to the seizure. Someone who has a seizure while working in the kitchen may have serious burns; someone who has a seizure while swimming may need emergency treatment after being pulled from the water; someone who has a seizure can fall and break bones. Fortunately, such events are uncommon. Most emergency treatment for epilepsy falls into one of three areas:

- first aid for seizures;
- treatment of status epilepticus;
- treatment for anticonvulsant drug overdose.

First Aid for Seizures

Some people who have lived with their seizures for years report that there is nothing more annoying than awakening in the emergency department of a hospital (yet again), having blood being drawn for anticonvulsant drug level determination (yet again) and being discharged home with nothing changed (yet again). In their case, a seizure is unpleasant but not an emergency requiring hospitalization. Other people

Knowing what to do

First aid isn't complicated, but it involves a sequence of actions and considerations that are beyond the range of this book. If you haven't taken a course in first aid and CPR (cardiopulmonary resuscitation) – or haven't taken one for years – it's time to sign up. Courses are available from many sources (check your Yellow Pages) and usually last a few evenings or a weekend. Ask a friend to sign up with you; you'll have a good time, and you'll end up knowing a lot more about emergencies large and small.

complain that they are neglected and ignored while they are having a seizure; some recall having a generalized seizure on a city street while passersby either stepped over them or crossed to the other side of the street. One woman had to cancel her credit cards three times in two years because the only people who paid any attention to her during a seizure in a public place were thieves who stole her purse.

What should you do if you encounter someone having a seizure? Use your common sense. Many seizure types – such as generalized absence seizures or complex partial seizures, which involve relatively brief episodes of unresponsiveness – don't require any specific first aid measures. The generalized tonic clonic seizure is the one that most frequently calls for some form of first aid.

First, forget the old myth about the person swallowing his or her tongue. There is absolutely no need to insert any object whatever into the person's mouth. In fact, doing so may result in tooth breakage and further complications to the seizure. Moreover, if you stick your fingers into the mouth of someone in this condition you may get your fingers badly bitten. The person may be turning blue but this is for other reasons; it's impossible to swallow your tongue.

During the seizure, try to make sure there is nothing within reach that could harm the person if he or she struck it. If the person thrashes about, don't attempt to restrain the actions.

There may be loss of bladder or bowel control. After the seizure, the person should be placed on his or her left side. There is a small risk of post-seizure vomiting, before the person is fully alert and aware, so the head should be turned so that any vomit will drain out of the mouth without being inhaled. Stay with the person until he or she recovers (5 to 20 minutes). The person will be a bit confused at first, but will gradually return to normal.

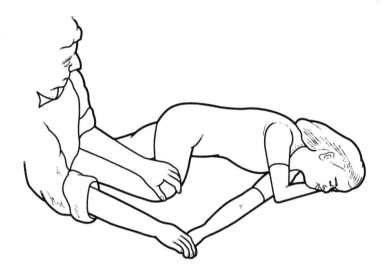

Someone who has never seen a seizure before often finds the experience frightening. People having seizures may turn blue or gray, and blood may come from their mouths. The blue or gray color (*cyanosis*) is the result of insufficient oxygen in the blood, because the person may have temporarily stopped breathing during the first few moments of the seizure. When blood comes from the mouth, it does not indicate life-threatening internal bleeding; the person has probably bitten the inside of the tongue or mouth. This is quite common during seizures.

What NOT to do

During World War I, a soldier, William, awakened in a field hospital with no recollection of how he had gotten there. Details were supplied by several of his comrades. He had obeyed an order to go "over the top" and had been advancing through no-man's-land. An exploding artillery shell had flung him high into the air, and in falling he had struck his head on a piece of wooden debris, and had been knocked unconscious. When he regained consciousness, he had severe pain in his tongue and his lip. There had also been bleeding, and he had the taste of dried blood in his mouth and over his lips. While lying in the mud of the battlefield, he had had a seizure. One of his comrades, imagining that he might swallow his tongue, had put a safety pin through his tongue and lip. After the war, William developed generalized tonic clonic seizures which continued sporadically throughout his life. During a number of these seizures he bit his tongue, but the pain of these tongue bites, he said, never came close to the pain of having a safety pin attaching his tongue to his lip.

Should you call an ambulance or take the person to a hospital? That depends. Some people experience three or four generalized tonic clonic seizures a month, and the last thing they want is a trip to hospital every time. However, if you come upon a stranger having a seizure, you may not be sure of the circumstances. Check for a medical-alert tag once the convulsions subside. Unless you can determine that the person is known to be epileptic, play it safe, and call for an ambulance.

In general, a seizure lasts from 90 to 120 seconds. If it continues for more than four minutes, or if the person has had more than two or three seizures in a half hour, seeking medical attention is probably appropriate.

If you encounter an accident scene in which someone has experienced a head injury and is having a seizure, it's important to stay calm and remember that the standard rules of first aid still apply. The seizure may appear dramatic, but it's not the problem – it's probably only a symptom of an underlying brain injury resulting from the accident. Furthermore, if the head has been injured there may also be damage to the neck, and that creates a risk of spinal-cord injury and paralysis. Avoid moving the person unless he or she is in *immediate danger* (from fire, for example). If you are trained in first aid, you know what else to do; otherwise, use your common sense and get help as soon as possible.

If you have a seizure disorder, it's a good idea to wear a medical-alert bracelet or neck tag or some other form of identification, indicating your condition and what medication you are taking. Such information is helpful to first-aiders and ambulance personnel, as well as medical staff in the emergency department.

Status Epilepticus
Someone who has a continuous seizure lasting more than thirty minutes, or who has multiple seizures continuing for more than half an hour without regaining consciousness in between, is diagnosed as being in *status epilepticus* (a continuous epileptic condition).

The characteristics of status epilepticus are variable, depending on the seizure type. It is generally classified as partial or generalized. Partial status epilepticus arises from either continuous or recurrent simple or complex partial seizures. Generalized convulsive status epilepticus is a true medical emergency.

Causes and Consequences of Status Epilepticus
The causes of status epilepticus are as numerous as the causes of seizures. Head trauma, meningitis, hypoglycemia, asphyxia, pregnancy complications, drug intoxication and drug withdrawal are all potential causes of both epilepsy and status epilepticus. Even chronic, progressive neurologic disorders, such as brain tumors or neurodegenerative disease, can account for status epilepticus.

The condition is found in all age groups, but tends to be somewhat more common in young children and in adults over the age of 60. Although it may develop in people with no history of epilepsy, most patients with status epilepticus have preexisting epilepsy, and the status epilepticus is precipitated by abrupt anticonvulsant drug withdrawal, significant sleep deprivation or some illness associated with either a high fever or an inability to take anticonvulsant drugs.

At 18, Paul had been experiencing seizures for four years: about six generalized tonic clonic seizures annually. The anticonvulsant drug he was taking, phenytoin, was not adequately controlling his seizures. Moreover, his gums were inflamed and they bled every time he brushed his teeth. He had developed significant acne. His girlfriend had made a number of hurtful comments concerning his physical appearance. One day, angry and frustrated, Paul flushed all his phenytoin down the toilet.

Ten days after stopping the phenytoin, he had a severe generalized tonic clonic seizure which had been going on for more than 20 minutes when he was taken to the hospital. His condition was diagnosed as status epilepticus. He was given 2 mg of lorazepam and 1 gram of phenytoin intravenously. (Lorazepam is a 1,4-benzodiazepine, like clonazepam. However, lorazepam can be given intravenously for seizure emergencies.) This failed to control his seizures. Next, he was given a large intravenous dose of phenobarbital. Because of the combined effects of phenobarbital and lorazepam upon his breathing, a tube was inserted into his windpipe and he was put on a breathing machine. He was transferred to the intensive care unit (ICU).

Twenty-four hours later, an EEG demonstrated no ongoing seizure activity. However, his stay in the ICU was complicated by severe pneumonia. Paul spent three and a half weeks in hospital before being discharged on phenytoin, 300 mg per

Can my seizures damage my brain and make my epilepsy worse?

This question – whether seizures beget seizures – is difficult and controversial. Neurologists and epilepsy researchers have wondered for years whether epilepsy is a progressive disorder. Many researchers believe that it is; many others believe that it isn't. At present there is no convincing evidence that the typical seizure, lasting one to three minutes, does any brain damage. Only status epilepticus, with its prolonged convulsions, appears to carry this risk.

day. Over the ensuing months this was gradually changed to carbamazepine. Although Paul has about four seizures per year, he now almost never misses an anticonvulsant tablet.

The consequences of status epilepticus can be severe. The risk of death is less than 8 percent in children, but some studies have reported an associated mortality rate of almost 30 percent in adults. Death is usually attributed to the underlying cause of the status epilepticus (such as head trauma) rather than the seizures themselves, but complications such as pneumonia can also occur, and a generalized seizure that persists for 30 to 60 minutes may itself cause brain damage.

Status epilepticus is generally a serious medical emergency. Your doctor will not waste time getting a CT scan or other imaging; these can be done after the seizures are controlled. You will be given lorazepam (or diazepam) and phenytoin intravenously. After 30 to 50 minutes phenobarbital is administered, also intravenously. Subsequent to this, pentobarbital may also be given.

Anticonvulsant Overdose

An anticonvulsant overdose is also a medical emergency. The symptoms of such an overdose, whether accidental or deliberate, are highly variable, depending on what drug was taken. Somewhat surprisingly, seizures are a very common symptom of an anticonvulsant drug overdose; these drugs suppress or prevent seizures at therapeutic doses, but aggravate or cause them at very high doses. Since anticonvulsant drugs are designed to enter the brain and suppress electrical activity, an overdose can lead to unconsciousness or coma; it may also interfere with the electrical activity of the heart, causing heart rhythm problems and, rarely, stoppage of the heart. The risk from anticonvulsants is quite variable; with some, such as gabapentin, the toxic side effects of an overdose seem to be less severe.

A close call

In mid-December, Barbara, a first-year university student, was brought into a hospital emergency department in status epilepticus. Since her friends said she had no health problems, it was assumed that she was experiencing the first seizure of her life. She was given intravenous lorazepam and phenytoin, and the seizures stopped.

Then the clinical chemist in the hospital reported toxic amounts of carbamazepine in Barbara's blood. This was totally unexpected. The emergency department physicians certainly had not given her any carbamazepine. Investigating further, the doctors learned that police officers had found a suicide note at her home. Barbara had tried to commit suicide with a deliberate overdose of carbamazepine.

Ultimately, the story unfolded. Barbara had been diagnosed with a seizure disorder approximately six years earlier, and had been taking carbamazepine. When she moved to a different city, she didn't tell her roommates that she had seizures. She was an outstanding student, at the top of her class, and under a tremendous amount of parental pressure to do well academically. She had applied for a prestigious physics scholarship; the winner was to be notified by December 10. When that day arrived and she had heard nothing, she assumed that she hadn't won the scholarship, and in sudden despair she swallowed the remaining 105 carbamazepine tablets in her pill bottle. Fortunately, Barbara recovered from her desperate act, and the letter stating that she had won the scholarship arrived the next day; her roommate brought it to her in hospital.

Take-home points

- Never, ever put any object into the mouth of a person having a seizure.
- Status epilepticus is a medical emergency that should be treated in hospital.
- There are many possible causes of status epilepticus, including the abrupt cessation of anticonvulsant drugs.
- An overdose of anticonvulsant drugs can actually cause seizures,

EIGHT

Seizures in Infants, Children and the Elderly

M any epilepsies and other seizure disorders appear for the first time in childhood. The later years – 70 and beyond – are also a time when the disorders are likely to commence; strokes and medication problems increase the likelihood of seizures.

The age of a seizure patient is relevant because children handle drugs differently from adults. Likewise, the elderly metabolize drugs differently from young adults. Your doctor will take these facts into consideration when prescribing treatment. Phenobarbital, for example, produces sedation in young adults. In children it can cause increased excitability, with an inability to sit still and concentrate, whereas the elderly are even more susceptible to the sedating effects than young adults, and frequently require smaller doses.

Seizures in Newborns
Seizures may occur in the first month of life. If the child was born prematurely, these seizures come at a time when the child,

in normal circumstances, would still be in the womb. Seizures in newborns can look quite different from the seizures of older children or adults. They are diagnosed on the basis of a variety of sudden or *paroxysmal* behaviors, including intermittent spells with no breathing, grimacing, sudden loss of muscle tone, repetitive twitching of the face or a single limb, bicycling movements of the legs, and lip-smacking or bizarre mouth movements. The particular behaviors reflect the newborn's stage of development, not the cause of the seizure.

The causes of neonatal (newborn) seizures are many. The most common causes are brain infection (encephalitis or meningitis), brain hemorrhage, too little sugar in the blood (hypoglycemia), too little calcium in the blood (hypocalcemia), too little magnesium in the blood (hypomagnesemia), too little oxygen in the blood (hypoxia) or some other inborn error of chemical metabolism.

These seizures are affecting a very young, developing brain, and their seriousness cannot be overemphasized. In various studies, the mortality rate of neonatal seizures has been reported as ranging from 20 to 50 percent. A neonatal seizure must be treated as an emergency. In treating such seizures, the physicians first ensure that the infant is getting enough oxygen. Any imbalances of metabolism, such as hypoglycemia or hypocalcemia, are then treated. To control seizures, it may be necessary to use medication such as phenobarbital, phenytoin or lorazepam.

Seizures in Children

Febrile (Fever) Seizures

Children up to the age of four often experience seizures when they have a high fever. These are generalized tonic clonic seizures. Typically they are benign and do not require specific treatment. (Due to concern about Reye's syndrome, ASA – aspirin – should not be used to treat fever in this age group.) Young children seem to have a lower threshold for febrile seizures; that is, a fever that would not trigger a seizure in an older person may do so in a child. Also, it is not so much the actual temperature reached, but rather the rate at which the temperature climbs, that triggers the febrile seizures.

If the seizures are prolonged or repeated, consult your physician. Prolonged seizures can cause some minimal brain alteration, and may predispose the child to develop complex partial seizures later in life. However, the typical febrile seizure *does not mean* that the child will go on to develop epilepsy.

Febrile seizures occur in 7 percent of children between three months and six years of age, with 90 percent of these happening prior to age three. Sixty percent of children have only one febrile convulsion, 30 percent have two, and 10 percent experience three or more. The risk of going on to develop epilepsy is 2 to 3 percent. Febrile seizures can usually be diagnosed on the basis of history and physical examination. In straightforward cases an EEG is not required.

Absence Seizures

Absence seizures generally start between the ages of four and ten. This disorder tends to run in families, and is somewhat more common in girls.

The seizures are in the form of unresponsive staring spells. There is no warning or aura. The child simply stops and enters a blank spell for five to fifteen seconds. During this time there may be some eyelid fluttering, or no movement at all. The child remains in his or her original position, such as standing or sitting. After the spell the child returns immediately to normal. There is no post-seizure confusion. These spells may occur several hundred times per day.

The absent schoolchild

Christopher is eight. For the past three years he has had spells, which have been particularly noticeable at school. He appears to be experiencing about 200 spells a day, but he himself doesn't always know when he has had one. All his spells are the same. There is no warning; he just suddenly stops and stares for five or ten seconds. After the seizure he returns to normal, with no confusion or disorientation; it is as if those seconds have simply been cut out of his life. If he plays hard and gets out of breath, the spells become slightly worse.

His pediatrician felt confident that Christopher was having absence seizures. An EEG confirmed the diagnosis. Christopher was started on valproic acid and had an excellent response. He has done extremely well since that time.

Absence seizures should not be confused with complex partial seizures; the latter are also blank, unresponsive staring spells, but they last longer and are frequently preceded by an aura and followed by confusion. Many people use the term *petit mal epilepsy* for both absence seizures and complex partial seizures, but this is incorrect. Petit mal is an old term for absence seizures.

If your child has absence seizures, you will certainly be concerned about school performance. It's not surprising that a child having 200 ten-second episodes of unconsciousness per day may have difficulties learning to read or add. Too often, these spells are dismissed as daydreaming or inattention. These days, however, many teachers know how to recognize absence seizures, and they are often the first people to identify the problem.

This disorder is relatively easy to diagnose. The seizures are worsened by overbreathing (*hyperventilation*). The EEG demonstrates a characteristic abnormality called a *three-per-second spike-and-wave discharge*.

This is a primary generalized form of epilepsy. Response

to treatment with valproic acid, ethosuximide or a benzodi-azepine is usually quite good, and most children's absence seizures tend to "burn out" sometime between the ages of 16 and 20. A number of children with absence seizures also develop tonic clonic seizures during their childhood years, but in most cases the epilepsy has disappeared by adulthood.

There are a number of seizure disorders which (unlike absence seizures) are unique to the childhood years. As discussed earlier, there is a need to distinguish between seizure types and epilepsy types. The most characteristic childhood epilepsies are benign rolandic epilepsy and juvenile myoclonic epilepsy (see Chapter 3).

The Ketogenic Diet

The ketogenic diet is sometimes suggested as a method of controlling seizures in children. This is not a diet that you should undertake to give your child on your own; you will need the advice and supervision of both a dietitian and a physician.

The ketogenic diet is very high in fat and low in protein and carbohydrates. It produces a medical condition called ketosis, which has been recognized since biblical times as beneficial for seizure control. The modern ketogenic diet was first introduced in 1921, and is an attempt to reproduce the chemical effects of starvation without actually depriving the child of the nourishment needed for growth. It is generally recommended for seizure control when anticonvulsant drugs have failed. This diet is so carefully controlled that even the sugar or starch contained within pills has to be calculated. Just as food is restricted, so too are fluids. All liquids are calculated as part of the daily fluid allowance.

Sticking to a ketogenic diet can be very difficult. It requires dedication on the part of the child, the parents, the physician and the dietitian. Nevertheless, the ketogenic diet is sometimes very successful in suppressing seizures, and this may make the sacrifice worthwhile.

There are a number of variations of the ketogenic diet. The main one is the MCT (*medium chain triglycerides*) diet. During the first two years, 80 percent of the diet is fat. If all is going well, the ratio of fat can be slightly decreased, permitting more calories to be consumed in the form of carbohydrates or protein. Some children find the ketogenic diet tasteless and difficult to swallow, and it may cause gastrointestinal difficulties.

Children on either of these diets must be followed very carefully. If you feel your child should be on one of these diets, consult your physician; do not attempt to improvise.

Very little is known about the therapeutic effects of the ketogenic diet in adults. It is traditionally regarded as a therapeutic approach for children only.

Seizures in the Elderly

People in their seventies, eighties and beyond develop epilepsy at a higher rate than people a few years younger, and the problem is becoming more widespread as the population ages.

There are a number of causes of epileptic seizures in the elderly, but by far the most common – applying to some three-quarters of seizures – is cerebral vascular disease resulting from strokes or brain hemorrhages. Alzheimer's disease and other neurodegenerative disorders of the brain are the second most common cause and brain tumors are in third place. Drug toxicity, kidney failure and liver failure may also account for seizures in this age group.

The physical exertion of a generalized tonic clonic seizure is hard on anyone, and in a frail, elderly person it can lead to painful strains and sprains. In some people, especially women with osteoporosis (bone thinning), it can lead to bone fractures.

Finally, the physical strain of a seizure stresses the heart, occasionally producing heart-related chest pain (angina) or even heart attacks in this age group. Seizures do not lead to strokes.

In general, seizure disorders can be easily suppressed in elderly people. However, great care must be taken in the selection and administration of anticonvulsant drugs. Older people tend to be extremely sensitive to the toxicity of anticonvulsants. Side effects of confusion, disorientation and tiredness are much more frequent in the elderly. Older people may already have diminished kidney and liver function, which makes them more vulnerable to drug toxicity. Also, they tend to use more prescription and non-prescription drugs, so there is a greater likelihood of interactions between the anticonvulsants and other medications.

At 73, Ethel has a long-standing history of high blood pressure, diabetes, obesity and angina. She is on many medications.

About two years ago she had a minor stroke. Although she recovered well, she was left with mild weakness in her right hand and arm. Approximately a year ago she experienced her first two seizures. They began in her right arm but rapidly spread to full generalized tonic clonic (grand mal) seizures. Ethel was put on carbamazepine, but this produced fairly marked dizziness. It was replaced by phenytoin, which also produced substantial incoordination. After a further seizure, she was tried on gabapentin. She has done well on this medication and no more seizures have occurred.

The side effects of medication are magnified by other difficulties common in older people. Someone with poor vision may take an incorrect dose; someone on a tiny income may take pills every second day, rather than every day, in order to save money; someone in the early stages of Alzheimer's disease or another memory disorder may not always remember to take the pills.

Take-home points

- In general, febrile seizures in children are not a significant medical problem, and they do not usually lead to epilepsy. However, unexplained seizures in a newborn are an emergency.
- Absence seizures can sometimes explain daydreaming and poor performance in class.
- Many children grow out of absence seizures in their teenage years.
- Special care must be taken to protect the elderly from the toxicity of anticonvulsant drugs.

NINE

Other Special Considerations

Since epilepsy pervades all aspects of the lives of seizure patients, there are a number of special situations and complications that deserve discussion.

Seizures and Pregnancy

Fertility is generally reduced by 20 percent in epileptic women, due to the effects of seizures and anticonvulsants. Nevertheless, they can and do become pregnant. Women with seizure disorders constitute approximately 0.5 percent of all pregnant women, and epilepsy can be a source of significant complications during pregnancy. Generally, the woman's greatest concern is the effect of anticonvulsant drugs on the developing fetus. Current evidence suggests that the rate of malformations in children born to mothers who are taking anticonvulsant drugs is two to three times that of the general population. These malformations often involve the heart, but may also include the cleft palate–cleft lip syndrome.

As a general rule, the risk of either major or minor malformations in the baby of a woman taking anticonvulsant drugs is 4 to 6 percent. In women without seizures and not taking anticonvulsants, this risk is 1 to 2 percent, about the same as the risk for women without epilepsy. For a woman with epilepsy, however, the risk of birth defects must be balanced against the risk of seizures, which can endanger both the fetus and the mother. The highest risk of drug-induced malformation is in the first four weeks of the pregnancy, when a woman may still be unaware that she is pregnant.

Various anticonvulsants bring different risks of birth defects. Phenytoin and the barbiturates are associated with a mild increased risk of developmental abnormalities affecting the fingers and fingernails. In addition, heart defects and cleft palates have been linked to these drugs. The use of carbamazepine during pregnancy has been associated with a 0.5 percent risk of spina bifida, an abnormality that involves malformation of the spinal cord or the bones enclosing the spinal cord. Facial and limb malformations, though rare, have also been associated with carbamazepine use. Valproic acid produces a 1.5 to 2 percent risk of spina bifida. Almost all of the traditional anticonvulsant agents can cause birth defects. Indeed, a so-called *fetal anticonvulsant syndrome* has been described. This rare syndrome includes varying degrees and combinations of malformations to the face, arms and fingers, sometimes with associated cardiac defects and short stature. However, this cluster of abnormalities has also been documented in the offspring of women whose seizure disorders were not being treated, and in women who did not have seizure disorders and used no drugs.

Early studies of some of the newer anticonvulsant drugs, such as gabapentin and vigabatrin, suggest that they are less teratogenic (involved in causing birth defects) than the older drugs. However, our experience with these agents is so far quite limited, and it is too soon to make any definite statements about their safety.

What about risks posed by the seizures themselves? Women who are considering pregnancy are usually reassured to know

Getting the right answers

Mary began to have seizures at around age ten. The cause of her seizures has never really been determined, though birth trauma is suspected. Over the years she has had many EEGs, some of which demonstrated left temporal "sharp waves" and some of which were entirely normal. No anticonvulsant drug treatment has ever given her satisfactory seizure control. Although she has settled on carbamazepine, she continues to have approximately three seizures per month.

At the age of 25, Mary had been married for two years and passionately wanted children. However, she was concerned about passing the epilepsy on to her babies. She decided to speak to her family physician. Telling her that epilepsy was a horrible disease, he advised her to "nip it in the bud" and give up her hope for children. This was very difficult for Mary to accept. Next she spoke to her clergyman, but he agreed that it would probably be better if the "curse with which she was afflicted" was not "spread to the next generation." Devastated, Mary resigned herself to a childless life.

However, Mary joined an epilepsy society and at a meeting two years later she asked a visiting neurologist to explain why women with seizures were advised not to have children. She was stunned to hear that there was absolutely no reason why she shouldn't have a family.

Mary consulted another physician, and soon started on folic acid at 5 mg per day, and discontinued birth control. She was concerned about birth defects induced by carbamazepine, but her new physician felt that, because of the frequency and severity of her seizures, she should stay on the medication throughout any pregnancy.

Some six months later, Mary became pregnant. An ultrasound examination at 17 weeks was entirely normal. A slight increase in seizure frequency during the second trimester was treated with a small increase in her carbamazepine dose, and she delivered a healthy baby girl at full term. The child is normal in all respects. Mary and her husband are thrilled, and a lucky child has loving parents.

that, although generalized tonic clonic seizures make severe oxygen demands on the body of the pregnant woman, the developing child is unaffected by a typical seizure. However, status epilepticus or prolonged seizures could result in decreased blood supply to the placenta, although this is extremely rare.

The effect of pregnancy on seizure frequency is unpredictable. About 50 percent of pregnant women with seizure disorders experience no change in seizure frequency, about 25 percent experience an improvement and about 25 percent experience a worsening of their seizures. If worsening does occur, it tends to be late in the pregnancy. Possible reasons include elevated estrogen levels, decreased levels of anticonvulsant in the blood and sleep deprivation.

A rare disorder associated with pregnancy, *eclampsia*, arises from swelling and small hemorrhages within the mother's brain, and can cause generalized tonic clonic seizures. The treatment consists of control of high blood pressure, control of the brain swelling, and control of the seizures, with magnesium sulfate. In resistant cases, phenytoin or diazepam can also be used.

It's wise for women with seizure disorders to consider their options *before* deciding to become pregnant. Anticonvulsant medications can be changed, simplified or optimized prior to pregnancy. Carbamazepine, or possibly one of the newer drugs, may be preferable to agents such as phenytoin or valproic acid. If there is a family history of spina bifida, valproic acid or carbamazepine should be avoided. Five mg of folic acid per day should be taken by any woman who is actively trying to conceive. Anticonvulsant levels in the blood should be monitored and adjusted as necessary throughout the pregnancy to help prevent worsening seizures. High-resolution fetal ultrasound is advisable at 18 weeks, especially in women on either valproic acid or carbamazepine. Amniocentesis (sampling of the amniotic fluid) to measure alpha-fetoprotein (a chemical in the fluid) should be pursued if there is a suspicion of spina bifida on the ultrasound. Oral vitamin K supplementation of 20 mg per day should be taken for the four weeks prior to delivery, to decrease the likelihood of bleeding or hemorrhaging in the newborn. If the mother has been taking barbiturates, she and other caregivers should be aware of the possibility of withdrawal symptoms in the baby after the first week of life. The child may be excessively irritable, and may have early problems with breastfeeding.

There is no reason for a woman with a seizure disorder not to breastfeed. Typically, the amount of anticonvulsant drugs secreted in the breast milk is too small to affect the newborn significantly. Some infants have been reported to be drowsy when breastfeeding from mothers on phenobarbital and other barbiturates, but this is not a serious problem. What is important is that a new mother with seizures should have support and help. Caring for a newborn, especially with middle-of-the-night feedings, is exhausting, and the resulting sleep deprivation can increase the possibility of seizures.

Seizures and Birth Control

Oral contraceptives are four or five times more likely to fail if a woman is taking anticonvulsants. Women who are taking these drugs should use an oral contraceptive with more than 35 micrograms of estradiol, and even then there is an increased risk of pregnancy. Certain anticonvulsants, including valproic acid, vigabatrin and gabapentin, are less likely to decrease the effectiveness of oral contraceptives.

Seizures and Alcohol Use

Alcohol is associated with seizures. This is quite significant since alcohol is the most widely used and abused drug in the world.

The influence of alcohol on an existing seizure disorder is poorly understood. In some people alcohol appears to make an existing seizure disorder worse, but this is uncommon. After all, as anyone who has ever been drunk knows, alcohol tends to slow the brain processes down. Not surprisingly, its depressant effect on the brain slows down the electrical activity that

Falling down drunk

At 41, George has a long history of alcohol abuse and has been in and out of treatment programs for years. Over the past five years, he has had several episodes of withdrawal seizures and the DTs (delirium tremens); all of his seizures have been associated with alcohol withdrawal.

Lydia, his wife, returned home one Saturday evening, having spent the day with her sister, to find that George and his friend Jack had been drinking heavily for "six or seven hours." Jack told Lydia that George had fallen several times. At that moment, George collapsed and had a generalized convulsion. Jack said that it was "just the booze" and that they should let him sleep it off. Although she suspected that this was true, Lydia was concerned enough to telephone for an ambulance. George had a second generalized tonic clonic seizure on the way to the hospital.

The emergency room physician was unable to obtain any meaningful history from George, who had had two major seizures and was unresponsive. A CT scan of his head revealed a collection of blood on the surface of the brain: a subdural hematoma. One of the times George fell that evening, he had suffered head trauma. A neurosurgeon drained the collected blood. Ultimately, George made a full and uneventful recovery. If this had been left untreated, though, he might have died.

contributes to seizures. Thus alcohol may in fact have a weak antiseizure effect. Consequently, seizures are far more likely to occur from alcohol withdrawal than from alcohol intoxication. A doctor treating a person who is drunk and also having seizures will not assume that the alcohol is causing the seizures; he or she will look for other causes of seizures, especially head trauma.

Alcohol withdrawal seizures characteristically occur after chronic, heavy alcohol use, but they may happen after only several weeks of drinking. Although the seizures tend to follow the abrupt cessation of drinking, they may occur if alcohol is only reduced, not eliminated. Most commonly, the seizures start 18 to 24 hours after the alcohol intake stops, although they can come as early as 7 and as late as 48 hours after. Typically, the person experiences a cluster of three to four seizures over a six-hour period. About 40 percent of people have a single seizure, about 60 percent have multiple seizures and about 3 percent suffer status epilepticus. Approximately one-third will also develop delirium tremens.

Alcoholics are three times as likely to develop seizures as the general population. Ten to 15 percent of alcoholics have seizures, of which 66 percent are attributable to alcohol withdrawal. Furthermore, approximately 20 percent of newly diagnosed epilepsy patients have alcoholism as their only risk factor. The development of seizures in alcoholics is also related to head trauma due to falls while intoxicated.

Alcoholics who suffer withdrawal seizures should not be treated with anticonvulsant drugs. However, those who have had head trauma and have subsequently developed epilepsy should be put on anticonvulsants. Unfortunately, if these people start drinking again they forget to take their anticonvulsants, and frequently go into status epilepticus as a result of alcohol withdrawal – even before they stop drinking.

Most people with seizure disorders do not abuse alcohol. Like so many people in our society, they like to socialize and enjoy the occasional drink. If you read textbooks too closely or listen to pharmacists too carefully, you may come to believe that you have to avoid absolutely all alcohol while on anticonvulsant drugs. It's true that in an ideal world people on anticonvulsants wouldn't drink, but in the real world it probably does no harm for a person with a seizure disorder, on anticonvulsant drugs, to consume one or two alcoholic drinks occasionally. Of course, if you are one of those rare individuals in whom alcohol worsens seizures, you obviously shouldn't be drinking. Also, some people taking anticonvulsants note that their tolerance for alcohol is greatly reduced, so they get drunk more quickly. Furthermore, frequent use of alcohol will "turn on" enzymes in the liver that speed up the clearance of the anticonvulsant drugs, so the level of the anticonvulsant in the blood will drop and the probability of seizures will increase. On the whole, though, a few social drinks probably do no harm.

Seizures and Diet

A great deal has been written about diets, nutrition, megavitamins and trace metals in the treatment of epilepsy, but these treatments are generally ineffective. A very few adults with extremely rare seizure types may benefit from special diets. For example, in the uncommon disorder known as phenylketonuria, people may experience an improvement in their seizure disorders if they are fed a diet deficient in phenylanine, and there are some people whose seizures respond to vitamin B_6. However, these cases are rare. Most adults with seizures will *absolutely not benefit* from avoiding phenylanine or from taking increased amounts of vitamin B_6. The ketogenic diet for children under 12 is discussed in Chapter 8.

Seizures and Illegal Drugs

Street drugs are normally taken to alter mood or behavior; they are usually designed to excite or stimulate ("uppers") or to soothe and tranquilize ("downers"). They achieve their effects by influencing brain chemistry. Not surprisingly, they may also influence seizures and epilepsy.

Heroin and related narcotics are dangerous when abused. Although their use is not directly related to seizures, people with seizure disorders under the influence of heroin often fail to take their medications. Abused in large amounts, narcotics can affect oxygen use by the brain and thus indirectly lead to seizures. Likewise, high doses of stimulants like amphetamines can directly produce a risk of severe seizures in people with no previous history of epilepsy. Amphetamines can also cause sleep deprivation, indirectly increasing the possibility of seizures, especially in people who already have seizure disorders. Cocaine, a brain stimulant, is a very dangerous drug that frequently leads to seizures; it also tends to constrict blood vessels, causing stroke, which leads to seizures. Cocaine abuse is unfortunately a frequent cause of seizures in young people. The role of marijuana in epilepsy is much more controversial. The drug does have antiseizure properties, but these properties are not impressive. Despite the wishful thinking of some, there is little to recommend marijuana as an anticonvulsant agent when compared to the drugs in current medical use. Marijuana use can produce significant side effects, and withdrawal from marijuana increases the likelihood of seizures.

Seizures and Violence

This is an area where myth and misconception have flourished, perpetuating ancient ideas associating epilepsy with insanity and violence. Every so often, movies or television dramas show us maniacal epileptics going on killing sprees. Nothing could be further from reality.

There is no convincing evidence to suggest that a person with epilepsy would ever deliberately attack anyone during the course of a seizure. Thousands of people have been videotaped having seizures; none of them demonstrated violence directed at anyone.

Ellen is 48. She hasn't had an easy life. As a child she was beaten severely by her mother; she suffered head trauma from these beatings and developed epilepsy. She had complex partial seizures of right temporal lobe origin. Many of these seizures generalized to full tonic clonic seizures.

By her teenage years, Ellen was also having problems with the law. She had been arrested several times for selling drugs, especially cocaine. An acquaintance, Jeannine, testified against Ellen in court, reporting that Ellen was both a user and a seller of cocaine. This resulted in Ellen receiving a long prison sentence.

Several months after her parole, Ellen took a taxi to Jeannine's home and stabbed Jeannine eight times in the chest. Jeannine died almost immediately. Horrified neighbors witnessed this event, and saw Ellen running away from the scene, covered in blood. She was arrested 20 minutes later. The arresting police officers noted that Ellen appeared confused and dazed, and spent much of her time sitting in the back of the police car, staring straight ahead.

At the trial, Ellen's attorney claimed that she was not responsible since she had completed this act while in a seizure. The prosecution insisted that the act had been deliberate. Both sides brought in expert witnesses to support their points of view. Ultimately, Ellen was convicted of murder. The medical evidence did not support the defense claim that her epilepsy was a factor. The truth is that seizures do not cause directed, purposeful violence.

It's true that people having prolonged complex partial seizures sometimes wander about and shove people who attempt to restrain them, but if they are left without interference they simply continue to wander, and show no inclination toward violence. Similarly, a person in a post-seizure state of confusion may push someone out of the way, but such violence is random, not directed, and is certainly not intended to hurt anyone. There is no need for any concern about violence from people who suffer from seizures.

Seizures and Dental Care

Like many other medical disorders, epilepsy can lead to dental problems.

First, seizures can damage teeth. Especially during the tonic phase of a tonic clonic seizure, the teeth may be clenched so hard that root fractures, cracked cusps, split roots or even fractures of the crown can result. All of these may produce pain, but some of them require dental X-rays for proper diagnosis. Even more traumatic accidents can happen: for example, if a seizure occurs in the bathroom, the person may strike his or her face against a hard object such as the bathtub, breaking teeth. Finally, during seizures people frequently bite their tongue or the inner surface of their mouth. In rare cases this leads to infections that can affect the gums or teeth.

Anticonvulsant drugs can also affect dental health. Overgrowth of the gums (gingival hyperplasia) occurs in 40 to 50 percent of people receiving phenytoin, sometimes as early as two to three months after the start of the medication. The only remedy is to stop using phenytoin, and it may be months to a year before gum overgrowth is reduced. Since the gums grow down over the teeth, food and other material can become trapped under the guns and on the surface of the teeth, causing decay and cavities.

There is good evidence that serious attention to dental hygiene decreases the likelihood of gingival hyperplasia. Careful brushing and the regular use of floss are essential, and twice-yearly dental checkups are advisable.

Seizures and Depression

In some people, seizures and depression go hand in hand. There are often good reasons for unhappiness. The loss of your driver's license or your job, the stress of not knowing when another seizure is going to occur, the social embarrassment of having a seizure in a public place – none of this is easy. Epilepsy is a chronic disorder; there is no pill to take it away. It's hardly surprising that *reactive* or *secondary* depressions are common. The severity of the depression is highly variable. Some people simply feel unhappy. Others have a full spectrum of symptoms, including tearfulness, loss of motivation, lowered libido, poor appetite and early-morning awakening.

For reasons that are unclear, Patty developed seizures at age 30. No cause was ever found for her epilepsy.

Her seizures proved very difficult to control. She was treated with phenytoin, phenytoin plus phenobarbital, phenytoin plus carbamazepine, carbamazepine alone, and carbamazepine plus valproic acid. None of these worked well, and most gave her side effects. In addition to this, she lost her driver's license. Since she worked as a traveling sales agent, she next lost her job. She and her husband lived miles outside the city, and without her driver's license she felt isolated and stranded.

Patty began to feel quite depressed. She lost interest in her normal activities. She was frequently tearful. She began losing weight. Anxiety awakened her early in the morning, and she would be unable to go back to sleep. She went to her physician and a reactive depression was diagnosed. Since Patty also had migraine headaches, she was placed on amitriptyline as an antidepressant drug (amitriptyline works against both migraines and depression).

Several weeks after starting amitriptyline, she had a significant worsening of her seizures; apparently the antidepressant was the cause. The antidepressant was immediately stopped. Patty's depression deepened and she made an unsuccessful suicide attempt by drug overdose. She is still having a difficult and unhappy life, but she is now managing to cope better, with emotional support from her family.

Many people find that psychotherapy, or even sympathetic conversation, solves the problem. That is, all they really need is someone who is caring and understands the difficulty of a life in which you never know when you are going to have a seizure and perhaps become unconscious. Other people require antidepressant drugs. Currently, these fall into two broad categories: tricyclic antidepressants (e.g. amitriptyline, nortriptyline) or selective serotonin reuptake inhibitors (SSRIs; e.g. paroxetine, sertraline). Unfortunately, both of these classes of drugs have been implicated in making seizure disorders worse, the tricyclic antidepressants slightly more so. However, the influence of these drugs on a particular individual is unpredictable. Some people show a worsening of seizures when they are on antidepressants, others show an improvement and still others show no change at all. If antidepressants help you, you should use them. If this results in a worsening of your underlying seizure disorder, appropriate measures can be taken to treat the worsened seizures.

A final wrinkle in this story is the possibility that anticonvulsant drugs, especially vigabatrin, may themselves cause depression. If a person has a history of major depression, vigabatrin can aggravate or reinitiate this problem. When the vigabatrin is stopped, the depression resolves. The capacity of vigabatrin to initiate depression in a person who has no previous history of depression is more controversial. Various other anticonvulsants have also been implicated in producing depression, but much of the evidence is based on anecdotal reports and has not been tested scientifically. It seems possible and even likely that barbiturates, which produce tiredness and fatigue, could also produce depression. Other anticonvulsants, such as carbamazepine and valproic acid, seem to be less likely candidates, given that they are sometimes used to treat depression.

Take-home points

- There is no reason why a woman with epilepsy should not become pregnant.
- You can take measures before and during the pregnancy to minimize the risks of anticonvulsant drugs.
- Most women with epilepsy who are on anticonvulsants have perfectly normal pregnancies and babies.
- Seizures are more commonly associated with alcohol withdrawal than with intoxication, even acute intoxication.
- Seizures are not responsible for deliberate or aggressive violence.
- Scrupulous dental care is very important for people who have seizures, especially those on phenytoin.

TEN

Epilepsy and Lifestyle

Epilepsy affects the biggest decisions of your life: where you work, where you live, how you spend your spare time and – in some ways – how you relate to other people.

Driving

The ability to drive is a sign of freedom and maturity in our society. A driver's license is often necessary not just for social well-being but for employment, and many people regard driving as a right, not a privilege. The data concerning the ability of individuals with seizures to drive are somewhat confusing. Some studies suggest that they are better drivers, because they tend to be more careful and conscientious. Other studies suggest that the risk of automobile accidents is almost twice as high for people with epilepsy as for the general public, and that the increased risk relates not only to seizures but to associated neurological handicaps and to the toxicity of anticonvulsant medications.

Laws concerning driving and epilepsy vary from country to country, state to state and province to province. Many people with seizure disorders feel that the laws are a prime example of the prejudice against epilepsy that exists in our society. Physicians in many areas are required to report patients with seizure disorders for suspension of their driver's licenses. However, no one thinks about reporting a person with severe angina or cardiac arrhythmias. Our society assumes that an elderly person with a heart disorder is a much safer driver than a young person who has a single nocturnal (nighttime) seizure every ten months.

If you are that young person, you may feel tempted to lie to your physician in order to keep your driver's license, or to plead with him or her to lie for you. However, most people realize the importance of reporting their seizures to their physicians and the appropriate regulatory agencies. After all, they know how they would feel if, because of a seizure, they harmed someone. In general, they appreciate that the laws are there not to punish them, but to protect others.

Ignorance of the law in your area – whatever it may be – is no excuse for breaking it. Just as physicians are often legally required to report any driver who has a seizure disorder, their patients also have a responsibility to tell the licensing authority about any disorder that might preclude the safe operation of a motor vehicle.

Are these laws fair? Not necessarily. Seizures vary widely in type, severity and occurrence. What about a person who has had only one seizure? Should this person's driver's license be suspended? What about someone who only has nocturnal seizures? Wouldn't driving during daylight hours be safe? What about someone who is seizure-free but whose anticonvulsant medications are being experimentally withdrawn? What about patients with simple partial seizures and no loss of consciousness, people who are quite capable of pulling off the road if they experience, for example, shaking in one arm?

It makes sense that people with general-class licenses should not operate a motor vehicle until they have been seizure-free for one year, whether they are on or off medication. It's also reasonable that people with professional-class licenses (drivers of school buses, taxis, gasoline tanker trucks and so on) shouldn't drive as long as they are on anticonvulsant medications, and shouldn't drive until they have been seizure-free for five years. On one hand, some people would argue that even a history of seizures should disqualify a person from ever having a professional-class driver's license, but this point of view is perhaps a little extreme. On the other hand, while someone who has had a simple partial seizure with no loss of consciousness may be safe to drive, seizure disorders that stay confined to simple partial seizures are relatively uncommon. Such a person does have an increased likelihood of developing complex partial seizures or secondary generalized tonic clonic seizures.

Whatever uncertainty there may be about driving and epilepsy, the laws regarding flying a plane are uncompromising. The occurrence of any seizure at all disqualifies a person from piloting an aircraft for the rest of his or her life.

Therapy dogs

A small percentage of people continue to have frequent, unpredictable seizures in spite of medication. Some of them are now protecting themselves through a remarkable ally: specially trained "seizure dogs" who somehow sense a seizure 30 seconds or so before the person collapses. They may be trained to press against you to warn that it's time to move to a safe place; they may refuse to go up or down stairs when a seizure is coming on. Some dogs will even bring a blanket and a cellphone as you recover. Researchers aren't sure how the dogs sense seizures. Some suggest that they pick up subtle changes in odor or electrical signals. Others insist that dogs are just more sensitive to slight clues in posture and movement. However they do it, these dogs bring a whole new dimension to "man's best friend." For information on therapy dogs, consult your local epilepsy association.

Employment

The issue of epilepsy and employment is just as serious as that of epilepsy and driving. Despite widespread public-sector and private-sector information campaigns, people with seizure disorders are sometimes victims of discrimination in the workplace. Sometimes employees are fired when they develop seizures. They are usually the first ones laid off during a company downsizing, despite the fact that most countries have laws to protect people from workplace discrimination because of epilepsy. The employer often justifies the action with the excuse that people with epilepsy present a higher risk of accidents, not only to themselves but to others.

Of course it's important to protect everyone's access to employment, but the rights of others are equally important,

The complication of liability

David is a lathe operator in a medium-sized furniture factory. For a number of years, he has had "funny spells" which start with a strange "rising" sensation at the top of his abdomen. During this time he is fully alert and aware, and the sensation precedes his spells by two to three minutes. He then enters a blank, unresponsive staring state during which he is unaware of his surroundings. Since he is concerned about losing a finger or a hand during one of these spells, he takes the warning sensation very seriously and immediately stops working at the lathe. He has two or three of these spells per month. He has no concern for his safety at work, because he always has time to back away from the lathe.

David is the best lathe operator in the factory, and he handles all the special orders. His employers are quite pleased with his performance and have never had any complaints. Recently, though, Dave innocently mentioned his spells to the plant physician, who realized that they were complex partial seizures and expressed concern over Dave's safety and over the company's legal liability. Dave is now very worried. He can't afford to lose his job; his wife is expecting their first child. His employers don't want to lose such a valuable employee, but they don't want him to be harmed at work and they certainly don't want to face any legal liabilities. No one knows what to do, and Dave wishes he'd never mentioned his spells to the company physician.

and obviously seizures can result in harm in certain workplace environments. Just as a professional driver can't work safely with an active seizure disorder, people with such disorders shouldn't work at heights or in other positions that would result in injury should they have a sudden loss of consciousness. As a result, people with epilepsy do have a higher level of unemployment. Various studies indicate a rate two or three times that of the general population.

Despite the potential hazards, it's important for people with seizure disorders to be employed. It's crucial for their financial independence, their well-being and their self-esteem. Many employers are quite understanding and flexible in accommodating their needs. After all, a motivated and hardworking employee is an asset, with or without seizures.

Education

School can be a very unkind place. A young person with a seizure disorder may be subject to ridicule from classmates, and occasionally the teachers aren't much better. It's true that

---

Dealing with ignorance

Noreen was 12 years old. For a number of years she had had spells during which she laughed in a bizarre, uncontrolled way. An MRI scan showed an abnormality called a hypothalamic hamartoma (benign brain tumor). She was diagnosed as having gelastic ("laughter") seizures.

Noreen was getting into trouble at school because of these uncontrolled fits of laughter. She explained to her teacher that these were seizures, but her teacher informed her that this was utter nonsense "since everyone knows epileptics flop about like fish out of water." Noreen's parents were outraged. They found it unacceptable that this degree of prejudice should exist within the educational system. Unfortunately, the school principal agreed with the teacher that it was preposterous to think seizures could cause laughter.

Ultimately, Noreen's seizures were controlled by lamotrigine plus clobazam. She switched to a different school, and became a happy teenager.

some students who have seizure disorders related to brain injury also have learning disabilities and speech problems; not surprisingly, they require extra time and attention. But it's also true that many people with seizure disorders have normal or above-average intelligence.

If you have a child with epilepsy, you know that your son or daughter can and should attend school, and that the teachers should treat children with seizure disorders as they would any other student. School attendance – even if your child needs special classes because of medical problems – can only have a positive effect on his or her long-term social integration. Local epilepsy support groups frequently offer educational programs to help students and teachers learn more about seizure disorders.

Recreation

A great way for almost any child to gain peer-group acceptance and achieve greater confidence is through participation in sports and athletic competition. Concerned parents may be doubtful, fearing that their vulnerable child will be subject to ridicule or incomprehension. However, a protective approach generally does more harm than good – although you should obviously use your common sense in helping your child select a sporting activity.

Swimming is not advised for people with uncontrolled seizures, unless one-on-one supervision is available. Horseback riding, gymnastics and bicycling are not usually suitable for people whose seizures involve loss of consciousness. Competitive team sports with body contact (such as hockey or football) or impact sports (such as karate or boxing) are also risky because any brain injury may lead to worsening of the seizures. Scuba diving, parachuting and hang gliding are all too dangerous. However, basketball and volleyball are excel-

---

Satisfaction versus safety

Elizabeth has had seizures throughout most of her life (she is now 17). She has two or three seizures, usually nocturnal, per year. Despite this, she has become a competitive cyclist; the best in her age group in the city, she has also competed at the national level, and now has hopes of representing her country at an international competition. She bicycles 12 to 18 miles (20 to 30 km) a day, six days a week, in the streets of the city where she lives. Although always supportive of her daughter's cycling ambitions, her mother is concerned that Elizabeth will have a seizure and fall from the bicycle, and perhaps get hit by a car. Elizabeth insists that she's safe and there's nothing to worry about.

When Elizabeth was younger, her mother had the right to insist she stay safe. Now that she is almost grown up, Elizabeth has to practice setting her own limits. She may become more cautious if she has a few scares, or she may just have a higher "comfort level" where risk is concerned. Either way, the next few years will not be easy for her mother.

---

lent team sports for people with seizure disorders. Tennis and badminton are reasonable choices, and track-and-field events are also suitable.

Relationships

People who are fearful of involvement in sports, thinking that the exertion may cause seizures, may also fear sexual activity. They have nothing to worry about! Sex does not increase the frequency of seizures in people with epilepsy, unless it is associated with significant sleep deprivation. Nor does abstinence improve (or worsen) seizures.

Emotional difficulties in a relationship can be stressful, and stress can contribute to the worsening of a seizure disorder. Stress by itself, however, does not cause seizures. Once again, if the stress is associated with sleep deprivation, an increase or worsening of seizures may be the result. Marital strife, separation and divorce are often associated with a temporary worsening of seizure disorders.

Stress and seizures

Emotional stress may worsen a seizure disorder, and for some people management of stress is more effective in combating seizures than increased doses of anticonvulsants.

The physical mechanisms linking stress and seizures may not be obvious or direct. When you are under stress, your sleep patterns may be frequently disturbed, and lack of sleep certainly affects the likelihood of seizures. Other factors implicated in "stress convulsions" are primarily related to the use of alcohol and drugs. Some people use alcohol excessively while under stress, and withdrawal from this increased intake may predispose to seizures. Likewise, some people use benzodiazepines (tranquilizers such as diazepam and lorazepam). As with alcohol, withdrawal from benzodiazepines can make seizures more likely. Antipsychotic drugs (e.g. haloperidol, chlorpromazine) can also lower seizure thresholds. Similarly, the use of certain antidepressants (like amitriptyline) can predispose to seizures.

Household Design

Is there anything you can do to make your home safer for someone who has a seizure disorder? Yes, there are many common-sense measures you can take. People who have poorly controlled seizures should probably take showers in preference to baths, because of the possibility of drowning. Similarly, houses with multiple staircases are less desirable for a person who has frequent and poorly controlled seizures; bungalows or split-level houses are preferable. Also, forced-air heating is preferable to exposed heating elements such as radiators.

Within a house, the bathroom is the worst place to have a seizure. It's a small room filled with hard objects (the sink, toilet and tub). Since it's usually used in private, a mishap may not be discovered for a while. The kitchen, too, is dangerous. The back burners on the stove should be used whenever possible. Saucepan handles should be turned inwards. Electric kettles should have an automatic switch-off. Microwave ovens are preferable to conventional stoves. Dishes and cookware should ideally be unbreakable. Floors covered with carpets or rugs are slightly better than hard ceramic, cement or wood floors.

There are many potential sources of trouble in the average house, and some are not as obvious as hard corners and sharp edges. For example, some forms of epilepsy are television-induced. These seizures usually occur in front of the television set, and are generalized. But these are uncommon, and only a very thorough EEG examination can prove their existence. The EEGs usually show abnormal photosensitivity: that is, a flashing or strobe light can induce seizures. Other flickering lights (such as on a Christmas tree) may also trigger seizures.

Take the time to walk through your home, room by room – including such areas as basement, garage and patio – and look for hazards. Are all the heating devices safe? Do any lamps pose a hazard? Are there sharp edges or breakable items that should be removed or relocated? By thinking over the "what-ifs" that apply to the particular seizures you're dealing with, you can help yourself feel safer and more confident.

Insurance

Unfortunately, people with epilepsy sometimes have trouble obtaining life, health or disability insurance. If you have had this experience, take heart; the situation is improving. Insurance companies that rely on out-of-date information and prejudiced assumptions about epilepsy are on the way out. Shop around; policies vary from company to company, but most companies will consider your application on an individual basis. Provide an assessment of your medical condition from your physician or neurologist. Factors such as seizure frequency, medication use, employment history, alcohol use and driving record will all be taken into consideration when your application is being evaluated.

If you are turned down, it's important not to become discouraged. Even if one insurance company rejects your application, another may gladly accept it. Be sure to get quotations from as many insurance companies as you can. Your epilepsy association may have useful advice about local companies.

Take-home points

- Every province and state in the U.S. and Canada has rules governing epilepsy and driving; it is your responsibility to know these rules.
- It is a violation of your rights to be fired from your job simply for having seizures.
- Epilepsy is not incompatible with excellent school performance.
- Some minor household modifications may improve the safety of a home for a person with seizures.

ELEVEN

Medical Problems That Resemble Epilepsy

Seizures are sudden neurologic events, but not all sudden neurologic events are seizures. Other conditions can give rise to what appears to be a seizure. The person may lose consciousness and may have convulsive movements, which can make a correct diagnosis even more difficult.

What can cause such an event? Three mechanisms can lead to an abrupt and dramatic neurologic problem:

- electrical events (seizures);
- vascular (blood-flow) events (syncope, or fainting; mini-strokes);
- psychological events (pseudoseizures).

Electrical Events
As discussed in Chapter 2, an abnormal electrical discharge within the brain may cause a seizure and thus an abrupt neurologic abnormality.

Syncope

Syncope (fainting), pronounced *sin-co-pee*, is a sudden episode of loss of consciousness due to a temporary drop in the blood supply to brain. The causes of syncope are many. It occurs in completely healthy individuals as well as in people with serious cardiovascular disease.

The most common type is *vasovagal* syncope, and it most often occurs in adolescents and young adults. ("Vasovagal" refers to the nervous system's control of blood flow.) Vasovagal syncope is usually triggered by factors such as the sight of blood, frightening news, or sudden pain caused by a relatively minor injury. These faints start with muscle weakness, nausea, sweating, facial pallor, sighing and yawning, and proceed to lightheadedness, a sudden loss of consciousness and falling to the ground. These steps can follow one another very quickly, leaving the person no time to sit or lie down. Sometimes, two or three seconds after loss of consciousness, generalized jerks or irregular shaking movements are seen. This is called *convulsive syncope*, but it does *not* mean that the person is having a seizure, or has epilepsy. Consciousness is regained very quickly.

There are many other, less common causes of syncope. For instance, disturbances of the heart rhythm can produce

---

The family secret

Anne-Marie is 19. Her maternal grandmother and one paternal aunt have adult-acquired epilepsy disorders. For the past several years Anne-Marie has had infrequent spells, which are more likely to occur if she is excited or warm, and only happen when she is standing. First she feels short of breath and flushed; then she falls to the ground unconscious. After a second or two, she regains awareness. Anne-Marie's mother was convinced that her daughter had inherited the "family secret." She was quite skeptical when a neurologist suggested that her daughter's events were not seizures but fainting spells.

arrhythmia-induced syncope. Syncope can also arise from respiratory or lung disorders; for some people, coughing or sneezing can produce a faint. People have been known to faint while "bearing down" or "grunting" during a bowel movement. (The process of bearing down is also called a *valsalva maneuver*. Coughing, sneezing and valsalva maneuvers all tend to increase pressure within the chest, which reduces the blood supply to the brain and causes the faint.)

Even when a fainting person has shaking or jerking movements, distinguishing between syncope and seizures is usually not difficult. A faint tends to begin with dizziness, air hunger and facial pallor, and the loss of consciousness tends to be preceded by a dazed feeling. A faint almost never starts when the person is already lying down. In seizures, however, the loss of consciousness is usually very sudden. In syncope the loss of consciousness usually lasts a few seconds at most; in seizures the loss of consciousness is usually 40 to 90 seconds. A person with syncope has a pale complexion with heavy perspiration; in a seizure a person's complexion is ashen or cyanotic (bluish). The muscle tone of someone with syncope is flaccid (limp), but someone in a seizure has rigid muscles. In fainting the eyes are frequently rolled upwards; in seizures the eyes are sometimes turned to the side. Tongue biting is exceptionally rare in syncope, but is fairly common in seizures. Loss of bladder control is slightly more common in seizures, although it can also occur in syncope. After a faint the person is usually not confused; after a seizure, the person is very frequently confused, sometimes for a prolonged period of time. After a faint, muscle pain and headaches are rare; they are common after a seizure.

Mini-Strokes and Minor Strokes
Since strokes involve the sudden onset of neurologic symptoms, some people mistake them for seizures.

Sorting out the symptoms

Larry is 62. He has had high blood pressure for more than ten years and is taking medication to control it. Recently he was diagnosed with diabetes, which is being treated with diet, exercise and oral medications. Over a period of three weeks he had four spells that began with numbness ("like a dentist's freezing") in the thumb and index finger of his left hand. Over the course of five to ten minutes this sensation of numbness gradually spread up his left arm. Sometimes it affected the left side of his face or his left leg. Rarely, the numbness was accompanied by clumsiness or weakness in the left side of his body. It lasted for about ten minutes and then gradually reversed. After one of the spells he had a mild headache.

Larry was deeply concerned about these spells. In an attempt to gather more information, he spent many hours on the Internet, consulting a wide range of websites. He was convinced that he was having seizures. He was also aware – from surfing the Net – that when someone his age begins having seizures, a brain tumor is a possibility. He was extremely worried.

Larry went to an emergency department and was subsequently referred to a neurologist. His neurologic examination was normal, as were his EEG and a CT scan of his head. He was finally diagnosed as having transient ischemic attacks, or mini-strokes. This is a serious medical condition. Further tests showed a 50 percent blockage of one carotid artery. Larry was placed on a single enteric-coated aspirin per day, and his spells of numbness stopped.

The signs and symptoms of stroke (see Chapter 2) can be as varied as those of seizures. This is not surprising, since the signs and symptoms of a stroke will depend upon which part of the brain has been deprived of oxygen. There are a number of well-recognized clusters of symptoms associated with certain types of stroke. Sudden loss of vision in an eye (like a blind coming down over the eye) is a frequent form of TIA, referred to as *amaurosis fugax*. Strokes affecting the cerebral hemispheres lead to weakness over one side of the body (*hemiplegia*). Strokes affecting the brain stem can lead to staggering, double vision, and numbness or weakness in the face.

It's not difficult to tell the difference between a stroke and a seizure. Strokes are associated with what are called *negative* symptoms, seizures with *positive* symptoms. Negative, in this sense, means that function is lost; someone with a stroke loses vision in an eye or strength in an arm or a leg. Someone with a seizure, rather than losing a function, acquires a dysfunction – for example, shaking of an arm or leg, or visual hallucinations.

Strokes and seizures can occur together. As explained earlier, seizures and epilepsy are symptoms, not a disease. Stroke, on the other hand, is a disease, and it can injure brain cells and thus lead to seizures.

Sleep Disorders

Occasionally, sleep disorders mimic seizures, but studies in sleep labs have helped to establish a clear distinction between the two conditions. Since certain seizure disorders are primarily nocturnal, these studies are quite useful.

One class of sleep disorders that can mimic epilepsy is the *hypersomnias*. These tend to produce excessive daytime sleepiness. For example, *narcolepsy* is characterized by sudden, overwhelming daytime sleepiness; the person feels an irresistible urge to sleep, and simply does so, for brief periods. Sometimes associated with narcolepsy is *cataplexy*, which involves a sudden, extreme loss of body tone that can superficially resemble a drop-attack seizure. Another cause of excessive daytime sleepiness is *sleep apnea*, which tends to appear in overweight men who have high blood pressure and snore dramatically. People with sleep apnea disturb their own sleep, so they too tend to fall asleep during the day. Interestingly, people who have both seizures and sleep apnea sometimes experience an improvement in their seizures once the sleep apnea is corrected, since sleep deprivation increases the risk of seizures. In general, distinguishing between seizure disorders and sleep attacks during the day is not clinically difficult, because someone having a seizure is more profoundly unconscious.

The *insomnias* are another major category of sleep disorders. *Nocturnal myoclonus* is a form of insomnia that involves sudden lightning-like jumps. Most people have experienced a sudden jump that reawakens them just as they are falling asleep; this resembles a seizure, but it's actually a sleep disorder.

There are also *paroxysmal sleep disorders*. *Sleep-related enuresis* (bed-wetting) is occasionally confused with the urinary incontinence associated with nocturnal seizures. However, if there are no other features to suggest that a seizure has occurred, distinguishing between enuresis and seizure-related urinary incontinence is relatively straightforward. Occasionally, sleepwalking or sleep terrors may resemble seizure disorders, but only superficially. (Sleep terrors are spells in which children awaken screaming with fear, night after night.)

Anxiety and Pseudoseizures

A pseudoseizure is an event that looks like a seizure but is not related to an abnormal discharge of electrical activity from the brain, and does not correspond to any structural or physical abnormality of the brain. Pseudoseizures are more correctly called *spells of non-epileptic origin*. However, the word "pseudoseizure" is widely used. In years gone by, pseudoseizures were sometimes called *psychogenic* – in plain words, faked.

What causes pseudoseizures? Occasionally, although not often, the seizure is intentionally faked. For example, someone who has been hit on the head and wishes to sue the other party may fake seizures. The seizure feigned by the bona-fide seizure patient Smerdyakov in Dostoyevsky's *The Brothers Karamazov* is a famous example of a fake.

Much more commonly, pseudoseizures are not faked but are subconscious reactions to stressful situations. Imagine this scenario: four people are standing at a bus stop, looking toward the street. A person sneaks up behind them and fires a shotgun into the air. The first person faints; the second one wets himself; the third person has a rapid surge in blood pressure; and the fourth falls to the ground and twitches, apparently having a seizure. Pseudoseizures can be an abnormal coping mechanism that appears in stressful situations, but this doesn't mean they are deliberately faked. Why some people develop them under stressful circumstances is not clear.

Pseudoseizures and fake seizures

Jerry took his car to an internationally franchised muffler shop, and demanded that the mechanic show him which portions of his exhaust system required replacement. While walking toward his car, which was up on a hoist, he tripped over a wrench, fell forward and struck his head on the cement floor. He didn't lose consciousness, but he received a good-sized cut over his left eyebrow, which required suturing in a local emergency department.

Ten days later, Jerry developed unusual spells of relatively violent shaking in both arms. At times the shaking was rhythmical, with both arms in motion at the same time. At other times his head also shook from side to side in association with the arms shaking. These spells tended to last five to ten minutes. After the spell he rapidly returned to normal, but he expressed concern about the implications for his health. Indeed, on three occasions he called his wife or co-workers during a spell, so that they could see the violent shaking of his arms and head.

Jerry said he was angered that a careless mechanic had caused this injury. He consulted a lawyer. The lawyer felt that it would be a wise first measure to see a physician. Jerry saw his family doctor, who referred him to a neurologist. His neurologic examination was normal. A CT scan of his head was normal; an EEG was normal; a sleep-deprived EEG was normal. Jerry had one of his spells while he was with the neurologist. He was diagnosed as deliberately faking seizures to win financial compensation, and he didn't get any money.

It's very common for someone to have seizures *and* pseudo-seizures. In this case it's not easy to tell a real seizure from a pseudoseizure, but it's extremely important to do so. Someone having pseudoseizures is spared the potential toxicities of anti-convulsant drugs, and can also keep a driver's license.

A number of clues can help your doctor distinguish between pseudoseizures and epileptic seizures. Pseudoseizures can occur at any age, but tend to be more common in younger people. They tend to be triggered by emotionally charged circumstances. The duration of an epileptic seizure tends to be

---

Seizures and pseudoseizures

Over the past 12 years, Sheldon, a university biology student, has had six seizures. Sleep deprivation or fatigue seems to increase the likelihood of his having seizures. He has responded well to carbamazepine.

On the two nights preceding his final second-year examination, he stayed up until three a.m. and got up again at six to study. An hour before the exam he had a generalized tonic clonic seizure and was taken to the local hospital. He was given a medical certificate to excuse him from the examination, and two weeks later wrote a make-up exam.

During his third and fourth year Sheldon developed pre-exam seizures on six more occasions. Sometimes these were associated with sleep deprivation; sometimes they were not. His parents witnessed one of these seizures and felt that it was substantially different from his previous seizures. His arm-shaking was peculiar, and his pelvis rocked forwards and backwards, which it had not done in previous seizures. His mother was concerned that Sheldon's seizure disorder was worsening. On the advice of a physician at the university health department, Sheldon increased his carbamazepine dose. The result was dizziness, fatigue and a worsening academic performance.

Sheldon was now depressed and upset. With another set of examinations three weeks away, his seizures became quite variable; some were like his original seizures, but others were bizarre. Since his spells were occurring approximately once a day, he was admitted to hospital for video EEG monitoring and more intensive investigations. Ultimately it was determined that Sheldon had a mixture of seizures and pseudo-seizures, the latter apparently brought on by stress. Once he understood his condition, Sheldon improved. He wrote a make-up exam three months later, and did quite well.

shorter (under three minutes) than that of a pseudoseizure, which may last five or ten minutes. Moreover, the outward signs of a pseudoseizure are frequently different: pseudoseizures are often associated with forced eye closure, pelvic thrusting, side-to-side head movements, crying and irregular movement of the extremities. Pseudoseizures tend to occur during the day, whereas epileptic seizures may occur day or night, and are slightly more common at night. Although urinary incontinence may occur in either seizures or pseudoseizures, it tends to be somewhat more common in seizures. The EEG is normal during a pseudoseizure *and* immediately after it. Frequently the EEG is abnormal in true seizures, showing spikes or sharp waves during the seizure and diffuse slow-wave activity after.

Take-home points

- Not all disorders that involve falling to the ground and shaking are epilepsy.
- Syncope, or fainting, is one of the conditions most frequently misdiagnosed as epilepsy.
- Mini-strokes are sometimes mistaken for seizures; mini-strokes involve loss of function (e.g., weakness), whereas seizures involve an *added* function (e.g., shaking of a limb).
- Pseudoseizures are sometimes misdiagnosed as epilepsy.

TWELVE

Looking Ahead

Seizure disorders are difficult to deal with, both medically and personally. They can cause unhappiness and even hardship. But the sporadic nature of seizures may also be a blessing; between these disrupting events, most people can live normally, or very nearly so.

Year by year, too, the chances for seizure control are looking better. We've come a long way from the licorice and pigeon dung foisted on poor King Charles II, and we're learning more all the time. In the future there will be advances in our understanding of the human brain and how it works. Coupled with these advances will be improvements in our techniques for designing and developing better drugs and more useful medical treatments. The technology for engineering drugs to fit perfectly into the brain's receptors is advancing decade by decade. There may come a time when we have "smart bomb" drugs that attack a seizure focus with pinpoint accuracy.

In the meantime, what can you do to improve the situation? As far as possible, don't turn the disorder into a deep, dark secret. Most people these days know a little about epilepsy, and are curious to know more, but they are understandably apprehensive about dealing with the unexpected. Wherever possible, be frank with friends, relatives and co-workers about your seizures, and about the ups and downs you have with medications. If they show interest, explain the electrical origin of the seizures, and tell them what they can (and can't) do to help. It's especially helpful to be honest with children who are old enough to understand. What you tell them about your problem will affect their attitudes for a lifetime.

After all, this is the twenty-first century. Surely, by this time, we should be able to recognize seizures as one of the common medical problems that we are well on our way to solving.

Some Drugs Used in the Treatment of Epilepsy

Generic name	Some brand names	Remarks
Carbamazepine	Tegretol	
Clobazam†	Frisium	not available in U.S.
Clonazepam	Rivotril	
Diazepam	Valium	
Ethosuximide	Zarontin	
Felbamate*	Felbatol	not available in Canada
Gabapentin	Neurontin	
Lamotrigine	Lamictal	
Levetiracetam*	Keppra	not yet available in Canada
Lorazepam	Ativan	
Nitrazepam	Mogadon	
Oxcarbazepine*	Trileptal	not yet available in Canada
Phenobarbital		
Phenytoin	Dilantin	
Primidone	Mysoline	
Tiagabine*	Gabatril	not yet available in Canada
Topiramate	Topamax	
Valproic acid (divalproex)	Depakene	
Vigabatrin†	Sabril	not available in U.S.

*Available only in U.S.
†Available only in Canada

Glossary

Absence seizure: often called petit mal seizure. A brief seizure (under 20 seconds) that can include staring, blinking and automatic gestures. Common in children with epilepsy.

Ataxia: staggering, unsteadiness. Common side effect of many anticonvulsants.

Atonic seizure: also called a "drop attack." Characterized by sudden loss of muscle tone. Person may fall or drop objects, or lose consciousness.

Aura: feelings or movements that are part of a simple partial seizure, and may precede a generalized seizure. An aura may include odd actions, visions, sounds, or feelings of déjà vu (the sensation of encountering circumstances or a place previously experienced).

Automatism: repetitive, usually purposeless motion performed during a seizure. For example, lip smacking may be an automatism during a complex partial seizure.

Catamenial seizures: seizures related to the menstrual cycle. Typically they occur several days before menstrual bleeding begins.

Clonic seizure: one that includes jerking movements in part or all of the body.

Complex partial seizure: one that impairs consciousness and affects only part of the brain. It may follow a simple partial seizure.

Computerized axial tomography (CT) scan: also called CAT scan. An X-ray technique that uses a computer to create a detailed picture of a cross-section of the brain.

Consciousness: state of awareness or alertness.

Convulsion: older term for a generalized tonic clonic (grand mal) seizure.

Corpus callosotomy: treatment involving cutting the corpus callosum, the band of tissue connecting the two halves of the brain.

Drop attack: *see* **Atonic seizure.**

Electroencephalogram (EEG): indirect measurement of brain electrical activity as recorded at the skin surface. Often used to help diagnose epilepsy.

Encephalitis: *see* **Viral encephalitis.**

Epilepsy: disorder characterized by recurrent seizures. Also called a seizure disorder.

Febrile convulsion: childhood seizure occurring when body temperature rises quickly during a fever.

Focus: the site in the brain where the seizure originates; also called focal point.

Gelastic seizure: laughter seizure, frequently arising from a tumor called a hypothalamic hamartoma.

Generalized seizure: one that involves the entire brain.

Gingival hyperplasia: gum overgrowth in the mouth. An anticonvulsant side effect usually associated with phenytoin.

Grand mal: *see* **Tonic clonic seizure.**

Hyperventilation: abnormally fast, shallow breathing. Used during EEG recording.

Ketogenic diet: specific high-fat, low-carbohydrate diet sometimes used to control seizures in children after other measures have failed.

Magnetic resonance imaging (MRI): scanning test that uses a strong magnet to create images to detect structural abnormalities in the brain.

Meningitis: inflammation or infection of the covering of the brain. May be viral, bacterial or fungal. May lead to seizures.

Myoclonic seizure: brief muscle jerk caused by an abnormal electrical discharge in the brain.

Neurologist: doctor who specializes in brain disorders and other disorders of the nervous system.

Neurons: nerve cells that communicate through electrical messages.

Nocturnal seizure: one that occurs when a person is falling asleep, awakening or sleeping.

Partial seizure: one that involves only part of the brain.

Petit mal: *see* Absence seizure.

Photosensitivity: tendency to react to certain types of lights (including flashing or blinking lights), which can trigger a seizure.

Positron emission tomography (PET): computer imaging technique that uses low-energy radiation to show brain chemical activity.

Post-traumatic epilepsy: seizure disorder starting one to three years after head trauma.

Seizure: sudden discharge of electrical activity in the brain that causes changes in behavior, consciousness or perception.

Seizure threshold: level at which the brain's electrical activity causes a seizure.

Simple partial seizure: one that does not impair consciousness and affects only part of the brain.

Spike-and-wave abnormality: EEG abnormality associated with a susceptibility to seizures.

Status epilepticus: seizure or series of seizures lasting over 30 minutes. A potentially life-threatening condition that requires immediate medical attention.

Stroke: abnormal condition arising from insufficient blood flow to the brain, or from brain hemorrhage. A frequent cause of seizure.

Syncope: fainting. Sometimes mistaken for a seizure.

Temporal lobe: part of cerebral hemisphere, located on the side of the brain.

Temporal lobectomy: operation to remove front part of the temporal lobe. Used to treat severe complex partial seizures.

TIA: *see* Transient ischemic attack.

Tonic clonic seizure: formerly called a grand mal seizure. One that involves stiffening of the body and muscle jerks. May require medical attention.

Tonic seizure: one that causes rigidity on both sides of the body.

Transient ischemic attack (TIA): mini-stroke lasting less than 24 hours. Sometimes mistaken for a seizure.

Viral encephalitis: inflammation of the brain due to a viral infection, which can cause seizures.

Further Resources

Organizations

(For information on local self-help groups, contact these organizations.)

U.S.A.

American Epilepsy Society
342 North Main Street
West Hartford, CT
06117-2507
(860)586-7505
Fax: (860)586-7550
info@aesnet.org
www.aesnet.org

New York Hospital - Cornell
Medical Center
Comprehensive Epilepsy Center
Room K619 - 6th Floor
525 East 68th Street
New York, N.Y. 10021
Tel: (212) 746-2359
Fax: (212) 746-8984
epilepsy@mail.med.cornell.edu
neuro.med.cornell.edu/NYH-CMC

Epilepsy Foundation
4351 Garden City Drive
Landover, MD 20785
(301) 459-3700
Fax: (301)577-4941
Toll-free: 1-800-332-1000
postmaster@efa.org
www.epilepsyfoundation.org

Canada

Epilepsy Canada
1470 Peel Street, Suite 745
Montreal, PQ H3A 1T1
Toll-free: 1-877-734-0873
Fax: (514)845-7866
epilepsy@epilepsy.ca
www.epilepsy.ca

Books

Devinsky, Orrin, MD. *A Guide to Understanding and Living with Epilepsy*. Philadelphia: F.A. Davis Company, 1994.

Epilepsy Foundation of America. *Brothers and Sisters: A Guide for Families of Children with Epilepsy*. 1992

—— *Issues and Answers: A Guide for Parents of Teens and Young Adults with Epilepsy*. 1991.

Freeman, John M., MD, Eileen P.G. Vining, MD, Diana J. Pillas. *Seizures and Epilepsy in Childhood, A Guide for Parents*. Second Edition. Baltimore: Johns Hopkins University Press, 1997.

Lechtenberg, Richard, MD. *Epilepsy and the Family, A New Guide*. Cambridge, MA: Harvard University Press, 1999.

Marshall, Elona. *Your Child: Epilepsy, Easy to Follow Advice*. Boston, MA: Element Books Limited, 1998.

Schachter, Steven C., MD, and A. James Rowan, MD. *The Brainstorms Companion: Epilepsy in Our View*. Philadelphia: Raven Press, 1995.

Index

Page numbers in italic indicate a figure or table.